USAMRIID's MEDICAL MANAGEMENT OF BIOLOGICAL CASUALTIES HANDBOOK

SEVENTH EDITION SEPTEMBER 2011

FORT DETRICK, MARYLAND

USAMRIID's MEDICAL MANAGEMENT OF BIOLOGICAL CASUALTIES HANDBOOK

SEVENTH EDITION
September 2011

LEAD EDITOR
Zygmunt F. Dembek, PhD, MS, MPH (COL, USA, Ret.)

Contributing Editors
LTC Derron A. Alves, VC, USA
COL Ted J. Cieslak, MC, USA
Randall C. Culpepper, MD, MPH (CDR, USN, Ret.)
MAJ Christine A. Ege, VC, USA
MAJ Eric R. Fleming, MS, USA
Col George W. Christopher, MC, USAF
Pamela J. Glass, PhD
LTC Matthew J. Hepburn, MC, USA
LTC Shelley P. Honnold, VC, USA
CPT Monique S. Jesionowski, AN, USA
COL Mark G. Kortepeter, MC, USA
MAJ Charles L. Marchand, VC, USA
CPT Vanessa R. Melanson, MS, USA
COL Sherman A. McCall, MC, USA
COL Julie A. Pavlin, MC, USA
Phillip R. Pittman, MD, MPH (COL, USA, Ret.)
Mark A. Poli, PhD, DABT
MAJ Roseanne A. Ressner, MC, USA
CPT Thomas G. Robinson, AN, USA
LTC John M. Scherer, MS, USA
Bradley G. Stiles, PhD
COL Lawrence R. Suddendorf, MS, USAR
LTC Nicholas J. Vietri, MC, USA
Chris A. Whitehouse, PhD

Comments and suggestions are welcome and should be addressed to:
Division of Medicine
Attn: MCMR-UIM-S
U.S. Army Medical Research
Institute of Infectious Diseases (USAMRIID)
Fort Detrick, Maryland 21702-5011

PREFACE TO THE SEVENTH EDITION

The Medical Management of Biological Casualties Handbook, which has been known as the "Blue Book," has been enormously successful - far beyond our expectations. Since the first edition in 1993, the awareness of biological weapons in the U.S. has increased dramatically. Over 190,000 copies have been distributed to military and civilian healthcare providers around the world, primarily through USAMRIID's resident and off-site Medical Management of Biological Casualties course.

This seventh edition has been revised and updated to address our understanding of medical management for diseases caused by threat pathogens. New material on the Laboratory Response Network (LRN), the use of syndromic surveillance in a biological attack, and contagious casualty care should prove useful to our readers.

Our goal has been to make this reference useful for the healthcare provider on the front lines, whether on the battlefield or in a clinic, where basic summary and treatment information is quickly required. We believe we have been successful in this effort. We would like your feedback to make future editions more useful and readable. Thank you for your interest in this important subject.

—THE EDITORS

Acknowledgements

PREVIOUS EDITIONS

Editors: CAPT Duane Caneva, Lt Col Bridget K. Carr, COL (ret) Les Caudle, Col (ret) George Christopher, COL Ted Cieslak, CDR Ken Cole, CDR (ret) Randy Culpepper, CAPT Robert G. Darling, LTC Zygmunt F. Dembek, COL (ret) Edward Eitzen, Ms. Katheryn F. Kenyon, COL Mark G. Kortepeter, Dr. David Lange, LCDR James V. Lawler, MAJ Anthony C. Littrell, COL (ret) James W. Martin, COL (ret) Kelly McKee, COL (ret) Julie Pavlin, LTC (ret) Nelson W. Rebert, COL (ret) John Rowe, COL Scott A. Stanek, Mr. Richard J. Stevens, Lt Col Jon B. Woods.

Contributors: Dr. Richard Dukes, COL(ret) David Franz, COL (ret) Gerald Parker, COL (ret) Gerald Jennings, SGM Raymond Alston, COL (ret) James Arthur, COL (ret) W. Russell Byrne, Dr. John Ezzell, Ms. Sandy Flynn, COL (ret) Arthur Friedlander, Dr. Robert Hawley, COL (ret) Erik Henchal, COL (ret) Ted Hussey, Dr. Peter Jahrling, COL (ret) Ross LeClaire, Dr. George Ludwig, Mr. William Patrick, Dr. Mark Poli, Dr. Fred Sidell, Dr. Jonathon Smith, Mr. Richard J. Stevens, Dr. Jeff Teska, COL (ret) Stanley Wiener, and many others. The exclusion of anyone on this page is purely accidental and in no way lessens the gratitude we feel for contributions received.

DISCLAIMER

The purpose of this handbook is to provide concise supplemental reading material to assist healthcare providers in the management of biological casualties. Although every effort has been made to make the information in this handbook consistent with official policy and doctrine (see FM 8-284, *Treatment of Biological Warfare Agent Casualties*), the information contained in this handbook is not official Department of the Army policy or doctrine, and should not be construed as such.

As you review this handbook, you will find specific therapies and prophylactic regimens for the diseases mentioned. The majority of these are based upon standard treatment guidelines; however, some of the regimens noted may vary from information found in standard reference materials. The reason for this is that the clinical presentation of certain diseases caused by a weaponized biological agent (bio-agent) may vary from the endemic form of the disease. For ethical reasons, human challenge studies can only be performed with a limited number of these agents. Therefore, treatment and prophylaxis regimens may be derived from in vitro data, animal models, and limited human data. Occasionally you will find various Investigational New Drug (IND) products mentioned. They are often used in the laboratory to protect healthcare workers. These products are not available commercially, and can only be given under a specific protocol with informed consent. For guidelines on the use of IND products, see Appendix L. IND products are mentioned for the scientific completeness of the handbook, and are not necessarily to be construed as recommendations for therapy.

Executive Order 13139:

IMPROVING HEALTH PROTECTION OF MILITARY PERSONNEL PARTICIPATING IN PARTICULAR MILITARY OPERATIONS

On 30 September 1999, the President of the U.S. issued Executive Order 13139, which outlines the conditions under which IND and off-label pharmaceuticals can be administered to U.S. service members. This handbook discusses numerous pharmaceutical products, some of which are INDs. In certain other cases, licensed pharmaceuticals are discussed for use in a manner (or for a condition) other than that for which they were originally licensed (i.e., an "off-label" indication).

This executive order does not intend to alter the traditional physician-patient relationship or individual physician prescribing practices. Healthcare providers remain free to exercise clinical judgment and prescribe licensed pharmaceutical products as they deem appropriate for the optimal care of their patients. This policy does, however, potentially influence recommendations that might be made by U.S. government agencies and that might be applied to large numbers of service members outside of the individual physician-patient relationship. The following text presents a brief overview of EO 13139 for the benefit of the individual provider.

EO13139

Provides the Secretary of Defense guidance regarding the provision of IND products or products unapproved for their intended use as antidotes to chemical, biological, or radiological weapons;

Stipulates that the U.S. government will administer products approved by the Food and Drug Administration only for their intended use;

- Provides the circumstances and controls under which IND products may be used.

To administer an IND product:

- Informed consent must be obtained from individual service members
- The president may waive informed consent (at the request of the Secretary of Defense and only the Secretary of Defense) if:
  - -Informed consent is not feasible
  - -Informed consent is contrary to the best interests of the service member
  - -Obtaining informed consent is not in the best interests of national security.

TABLE OF CONTENTS

INTRODUCTION

Medical defense against the use of pathogens and toxins as weapons or terrorism is a subject previously unfamiliar to many healthcare providers. The U.S. military has performed ongoing research against biological weapon threats since World War II, but the terrorist attacks on the U.S. mainland in September 2001 and the anthrax mail attacks in October 2001 provided a wake-up call for lawmakers, the public at large, and medical providers of all backgrounds that the threat of biological attacks was real and required planning, training, and resources for response. There has been a consequent increase of interest among healthcare practitioners to understand better how to manage the medical consequences of exposure to biological weapons that can lead to mass casualties.

Numerous measures to improve preparedness for and response to biological warfare or bioterrorism are ongoing at local, state, and federal levels. Training efforts have increased in both military and civilian sectors. A week-long Medical Management of Chemical and Biological Casualties Course taught at both USAMRIID and USAMRICD trains hundreds of military and civilian medical professionals each year on biological and chemical medical defense. The highly successful USAMRIID international satellite, online, and DVD courses on the Medical Management of Biological Casualties have reached over hundreds of thousands of medical personnel since 1997.

Through this handbook and related courses, medical professionals learn about effective available medical countermeasures against many of the bacteria, viruses, and toxins that might be used as biological weapons against our military forces or civilian communities. The importance of this education cannot be overemphasized and it is hoped that healthcare professionals will develop a solid understanding of the biological threats we face and the effective medical defenses against these threats.

The global threat of the use of biological weapons is serious, and the potential for devastating casualties is high. There are many countries around the world suspected to have offensive biological weapons programs. However, with early recognition, intervention, and appropriate use of medical countermeasures either already developed or under development, many casualties can be prevented or minimized.

The purpose of this handbook is to serve as a concise, pocket-sized manual that can be pulled off the shelf (or from a pocket) in a crisis to guide medical personnel in the prophylaxis and management of biological casualties. It is designed as a quick reference and overview, and is not intended as a definitive text. A greater in-depth discussion of the agents covered here may be found in Army Surgeon General's Borden Institute Textbook of Military Medicine, "Medical Aspects of Biological Warfare" (2007) and in relevant infectious disease, tropical medicine, and disaster management textbooks.

HISTORY OF BIOLOGICAL WARFARE AND CURRENT THREAT

The use of biological weapons in warfare has been recorded throughout history. During the 12th –15th centuries BC, the Hittites are known to have driven diseased animals and people into enemy territory with the intent of initiating an epidemic. In the 6th century BC, the Assyrians poisoned enemy wells with rye ergot, and Greek general Solon used the herb hellebore to poison the water source of the city of Krissa during his siege. In 1346, plague broke out in the Tartar army during its siege of Kaffa (at present day Feodosia in the Crimea). The attackers hurled the corpses of plague victims over the city walls. Subsequently, the "Black Death" plague pandemic, spread throughout Europe and is thought to have caused the death of one-third of the population of Europe – as many as 25 million people. In 1422, at the siege of Karlstejn during the Hussite Wars in Bohemia, Prince Coribut hurled corpses of plague-stricken soldiers at the enemy troops, and Russian forces may have used the same tactic against the Swedes in 1710.

In 1611 in Jamestown Colony in Virginia, a toxic hallucinogenic drug derived from plants was used against the English settlers by Chief Powhatan. On several occasions throughout history, smallpox was used as a biological weapon. Pizarro is said to have presented South American natives with *Variola* virus-contaminated clothing in the 16th century. The English followed suit in 1763 when Sir Jeffery Amherst recommended that his troops to provide Indians loyal to the French with smallpox-laden blankets towards the close of the French and Indian War. Captain Simeon Ecuyer, one of Amherst's subordinates, gave blankets and a handkerchief from a smallpox hospital to Native Americans, after which he wrote: "I hope it will have the desired effect." Soon afterward, Native Americans defending Fort Carillon (now known as Fort Ticonderoga) sustained epidemic casualties, which directly contributed to the loss of the fort to the English. General George Washington ordered variolation (a precursor of smallpox vaccination, using material obtained from smallpox scabs) for the Continental Army in 1777 after the loss of the siege of Quebec, in part due to devastation rendered on his forces by smallpox, and because of concerns for purposeful spread of smallpox among the colonials by the British.

Use of biological weapons continued into the 1900s; however, the stakes became higher as the science of microbiology allowed for a new level of sophistication in producing agents. During World War I, German agents inoculated horses and cattle with anthrax and glanders at the Port of Baltimore before the animals were shipped to France. In 1937, Japan started an ambitious biowarfare program, located 40 miles south of Harbin, Manchuria, code-named "Unit 731." Studies directed by Japanese general and physician Shiro Ishii continued there until it was destroyed in 1945. A post-World War II investigation revealed that the Japanese researched numerous organisms and used prisoners of war as research subjects. About 1,000 human autopsies apparently were carried out at Unit 731, mostly on victims exposed to aerosolized anthrax. Many more prisoners and Chinese nationals may have died in this facility, up to 3,000 deaths. The Japanese also apparently used bio-agents in the field: after reported overflights by Japanese planes suspected of dropping plague-infected fleas, plague epidemics ensued in China and Manchuria, with resulting untold thousands of deaths. By 1945, the Japanese program had stockpiled 400 kilograms of anthrax to be used in a specially designed fragmentation bomb.

In 1942, the U.S. began its own research and development program in the use of bio-agents for offensive purposes. Similar programs existed in Canada, the United Kingdom (UK), and probably several other countries. This work was started, interestingly enough, in response to a perceived German biowarfare threat as opposed to a Japanese one. The U.S. research program was headquartered at Camp Detrick (now Fort Detrick), and produced agents and conducted field testing at other sites until 1969, when President Nixon stopped all offensive biological and toxin weapon research and production by executive order. Between May 1971 and May 1972, all stockpiles of bio-agents and munitions from the now defunct U.S. program were destroyed in the presence of monitors representing the U.S. Department of Agriculture, the Department of Health, Education, and Welfare, (now Health and Human Services), and the states of Arkansas, Colorado, and Maryland. Included among the bio-agents destroyed were *Bacillus anthracis*, botulinum toxin, *Francisella tularensis, Coxiella burnetii*, Venezuelan equine encephalitis virus, *Brucella suis*, and staphylococcal enterotoxin B. The U.S. Army began a medical defensive program in 1953 that continues today at USAMRIID.

In 1972, the U.S., UK, and USSR signed the Convention on the Prohibition of the Development, Production and Stockpiling of Bacteriological and Toxin Weapons and on Their Destruction, commonly called the Biological Weapons Convention. Over 140 countries have since added their ratification. This treaty prohibits the stockpiling of bio-agents for offensive military purposes, and also forbids research on agents for other than peaceful purposes. To strengthen efforts to combat the BW threat, signatory states agreed in November 2002 to have experts meet annually through 2006 to discuss and promote common understanding and effective action on biosecurity, national implementation measures, suspicious outbreaks of disease, disease surveillance, and codes of conduct for scientists. However, despite this historic agreement among nations, biowarfare research continued to flourish in many countries hostile to the U.S. Moreover, there have been several cases of suspected or actual release of biological weapons. Among the most notorious of these were the "yellow rain" incidents in Southeast Asia, the use of ricin as an assassination weapon in London in 1978, and the accidental release of weaponized anthrax spores at Sverdlovsk in 1979.

Testimony from the late 1970s indicated that Laos and Kampuchea were attacked by planes and helicopters delivering colored aerosols. After being exposed, people and animals became disoriented and ill, and a small percentage of those stricken died. Some of these clouds may have been comprised of trichothecene toxins (in particular, T2 mycotoxin). These attacks are grouped under the label "yellow rain." There has been a great deal of controversy about whether these clouds were truly biowarfare agents (bio-agents). Some have argued that the clouds were nothing more than feces produced by swarms of bees.

In 1978, Georgi Markov, a Bulgarian defector living in the UK, was attacked in London with a device disguised as an umbrella, which injected a tiny pellet filled with ricin toxin into the subcutaneous tissue of his leg. He died several days later. On autopsy, the tiny pellet was found and determined to contain ricin toxin. It was later revealed that the Bulgarian secret service carried out the assassination, and the technology to commit the crime was developed and supplied by the Soviet Union's secret service (KGB). Interestingly, never-used research conducted in the United States during the World War 1 revealed that ricin toxin-coated bullets produced shrapnel that caused fatal wounds.

In April, 1979, an incident occurred in Sverdlovsk (now Yekaterinburg) in the Soviet Union which appeared to be an accidental aerosol release of *Bacillus anthracis* spores from a Soviet military microbiology facility: Compound 19. At least 77 residents living downwind from this compound developed high fever and had difficulty breathing; a minimum of 66 cases died. The Soviet Ministry of Health blamed the deaths on the consumption of contaminated meat, and for years, controversy raged in the press over the actual cause of the outbreak. All evidence available to the United States government indicated a release of aerosolized *B. anthracis* spores. In the summer of 1992, U.S. intelligence officials were proven correct when the new Russian President, Boris Yeltsin, acknowledged that the Sverdlovsk incident was in fact related to military developments at the microbiology facility. In 1994, Harvard Professor Mathew Meselson and colleagues published an in-depth analysis of the Sverdlovsk incident. They documented that all of the cases from 1979 occurred within a narrow zone extending 4 kilometers downwind in a southeasterly direction from Compound 19. A more recently reported incident from the Soviet Union revealed that in 1971, a field test of smallpox biological weapon near Aralsk, Kazakhstan caused an outbreak of at least 10 cases and 1 death. In both Sverdlovsk and Aralsk, a massive intervention by public health authorities greatly helped to lower potential disease spread and deaths.

In August, 1991, the United Nations (UN) carried out its first inspection of Iraq's biowarfare capabilities in the aftermath of the Gulf War. On August 2, 1991, representatives of the Iraqi government announced to leaders of U.N. Special Commission Team 7 that they had conducted research into the offensive use of *B. anthracis*, botulinum toxins, and *Clostridium perfringens* (presumably one of its toxins), and other bio-agents. This open admission of biological weapons research verified many of the concerns of the U.S. intelligence community. Iraq had extensive and redundant research facilities at Salman Pak and other sites, many of which were destroyed during the war.

In 1995, further information on Iraq's offensive program was made available to UN inspectors. Iraq conducted research and development work on anthrax, botulinum toxins, *Clostridium perfringens*, aflatoxins, wheat cover smut, and ricin. Field trials were conducted with *B. subtilis* (a simulant for anthrax), botulinum toxin, and aflatoxin. Bio-agents were tested in various delivery systems, including rockets, aerial bombs, and spray tanks. In

December 1990, the Iraqis filled 100 R400 bombs with botulinum toxin, 50 with anthrax, and 16 with aflatoxin. In addition, 13 Al Hussein (SCUD) warheads were filled with botulinum toxin, 10 with anthrax, and 2 with aflatoxin. These weapons were deployed in January 1991 to four locations. In all, Iraq produced 19,000 liters of concentrated botulinum toxin (nearly 10,000 liters filled into munitions), 8,500 liters of concentrated anthrax (6,500 liters filled into munitions) and 2,200 liters of aflatoxin (1,580 liters filled into munitions). It appears that any subsequent biological weapons program in Iraq was limited to research.

According to many experts, the threat of biowarfare has increased in recent decades, with a number of countries working on the offensive use of these agents. The extensive program of the former Soviet Union is now primarily under the control of Russia. Former Russian president Boris Yeltsin stated that he would put an end to further offensive biological research; however, the degree to which the program was scaled back is not known. Revelations from Ken Alibek, a senior biowarfare program manager who defected from Russia in 1992, outlined a remarkably robust biowarfare program, which included active research into genetic engineering, binary bioagents and chimeras, and capacity to produce industrial quantities of agents. There is also growing concern that the smallpox virus, lawfully stored in only two laboratories at the Centers for Disease Control and Prevention (CDC) in Atlanta and the Russian State Centre for Research on Virology and Biotechnology (Vektor), may exist in other countries around the globe.

There is intense concern in the west about the possibility of proliferation or enhancement of offensive programs in countries hostile to the law-abiding democracies, due to the potential hiring of expatriate Russian scientists. Iran and Syria have been identified as countries "aggressively seeking" nuclear, biological, and chemical weapons. Libya was also included; however, in 2003 Libya has renounced further pursuit of offensive programs.

The 1990s saw increasing concern over the possibility of the terrorist use of bio-agents to threaten either military or civilian populations. Extremist groups have tried to obtain microorganisms that could be used as biological weapons. The 1995 sarin nerve agent attack in the Tokyo subway system raised awareness that terrorist organizations could potentially acquire or develop weapons of mass destruction (WMD) for use against civilian populations. Subsequent investigations revealed that, on several occasions, the Aum Shinrikyo cult had attempted to release botulinum toxin (1993 and 1995) and *B. anthracis* (1995) from trucks and rooftops. Fortunately, these efforts were unsuccessful. The Department of Defense initially led a federal effort to train the first responders in 120 American cities to be prepared to act in case of a domestic terrorist incident involving WMD. This program was subsequently handed over to the Department of Justice, and then to the Department of Homeland Security (DHS). First responders, public health and medical personnel, and law enforcement agencies have dealt with the exponential increase in biological weapons hoaxes around the country over the past several years.

The events of September 11, 2001, and subsequent anthrax mail attacks brought immediacy to planning for the terrorist use of WMD in the U.S. Anthrax-laden letters placed in the mail caused 23 probable or confirmed cases of anthrax-related illness and five deaths, mostly among postal workers and those handling mail. On October 17, 2001, U.S. lawmakers were directly affected by anthrax contamination leading to closure of the Hart Senate Office Building in Washington, D.C. Terrorist plots to use ricin were uncovered in England in January, 2003. Ricin was also found in a South Carolina postal facility in October, 2003 and the Dirksen Senate Office Building in Washington, D.C. in February, 2004. Ricin incidents continue to occur due to the ready availability of the source material from castor beans.

The National Strategy for Homeland Security and the Homeland Security Act of 2002 were developed in response to the terrorist attacks. The Department of Homeland Security (DHS), with over 180,000 personnel, was established to provide the unifying foundation for a national network of organizations and institutions involved in efforts to secure the nation. Over $8 billion from the DHS has been awarded since March, 2003 to help first responders and state and local governments to prevent, respond to and recover from potential acts of terrorism and other disasters. The Office for Domestic Preparedness (ODP) is the principal component of the DHS responsible for preparing the U.S. for acts of terrorism by providing training, funds for the purchase of equipment, support for the planning and execution of exercises, technical assistance and other support to assist states and local jurisdictions to prevent, plan for, and respond to acts of terrorism.

The Public Health Security and Bioterrorism Response Act of 2002 requires drinking water facilities to conduct vulnerability assessments; all universities and laboratories that work with biological material that could pose a public-health threat have to be registered with the U.S. Department of Health and Human Services or the U.S. Department of Agriculture; and new steps were imposed to limit access to various biological threat agents. Smallpox preparedness was implemented, including a civilian vaccination program, vaccine injury compensation program, and aid to the states. Before the March 2003 invasion of Iraq, state and local health departments and hospitals nationwide conducted smallpox vaccinations of healthcare workers and have since developed statewide bioterrorism response plans.

The threat of the use of biological weapons against U.S. military forces and civilians may be more acute than at any time in U.S. history, due to the widespread availability of agents, along with knowledge of production methodologies and potential dissemination devices. Therefore, awareness of and preparedness for this threat will require the education of our government officials, healthcare providers, public health officials, and law enforcement personnel and is vital to our national security.

DISTINGUISHING BETWEEN NATURAL AND INTENTIONAL DISEASE OUTBREAKS

The ability to determine who is at risk and to make appropriate decisions regarding prophylaxis and other response measures after a biological attack, (whether from bioterrorism or biological warfare on the battlefield), will require the tools of epidemiology. After a successful covert attack, the most likely first indicator will be increased numbers of patients presenting to individual healthcare providers or emergency departments with similar clinical features, caused by the disseminated disease agent. The possibility exists that other medical professionals, such as pharmacists or laboratorians, who may receive more than the usual numbers of prescriptions or requests for laboratory tests may be the first to recognize that something unusual is occurring. Because animals may be sentinels of disease in humans and many of the high-threat bioagents discussed in this book are zoonoses, it is possible that veterinarians might recognize an event in animals before it is recognized in humans. Medical examiners, coroners, and non-medical professionals, such as morticians, may also be important sentinel event reporters.

To help ensure a prompt and efficient response, public health authorities must implement surveillance systems so they know the background disease rates and can recognize patterns of nonspecific syndromes that could indicate the early manifestations of a bioagent attack. The system must be timely, sensitive, specific, and practical. To recognize any unusual changes in disease occurrence, surveillance of background disease activity should be ongoing, and any variation should be followed up promptly with a directed examination of the facts regarding the change. In the past several years, many public health authorities have initiated syndrome-based surveillance systems in an attempt to achieve near real-time detection of unusual events. Regardless of the system, a sudden sharp increase in illness rates, or the diagnosis of a rare or unusual illness may still be first recognized by clinicians or laboratorians.

After detection of a potential disease outbreak, whether natural or human-engineered, a thorough epidemiological investigation will assist medical personnel in identifying the pathogen and lead to the institution of appropriate medical interventions. Identifying the affected population, possible routes of exposure, signs and symptoms of disease, along with rapid laboratory identification of the causative agent(s), will greatly increase the ability to institute an appropriate medical and public health response. Good epidemiologic information can guide the appropriate follow-up of those potentially exposed, as well as assist in risk communication and responses to the media.

Many diseases caused by weaponized bio-agents present with nonspecific clinical features that may be difficult to diagnose and recognize as a biological attack. Features of the epidemic may be important in differentiating between a natural and a terrorist or warfare attack. Epidemiologic clues that may indicate an intentional attack are listed in Table 1. While a helpful guide, it is important to remember that naturally occurring epidemics may have one or more of these characteristics and a biological attack may have none. However, if many of the listed clues are recognized, one's index of suspicion for an intentionally spread outbreak should increase.

Once a biological attack or any outbreak of disease is suspected, the epidemiologic investigation should begin. There are some important differences between epidemiological investigations for natural and deliberate outbreaks. Because the use of a biological weapon is a criminal act, it will be very important for the evidence gathered to be able to stand up to scrutiny in court. Therefore, if suspected to be intentional, samples must be handled through a chain of custody and there must be good communication and information sharing between public health and law-enforcement authorities. In addition, because the attack may be intentional, one must be prepared for the unexpected – there is the possibility of multiple outbreaks at different locations as well as the use of multiple different agents, including mixed chemical and bio-agents or multiple bio-agents.

The first step in the investigation is to confirm that a disease outbreak has occurred. Because an outbreak has a higher rate of an illness than is normally seen in a specific population, it is helpful to have background surveillance data to determine if what is being seen constitutes a deviation from the norm. For example, in mid-winter, thousands of cases of influenza may not be considered an outbreak, whereas in the summer, it might be highly unusual. In addition, even a single case of a very unusual illness, such as inhalational anthrax, might constitute an outbreak and should be viewed with suspicion. The clinical features seen in the initial cases can be used to construct a case definition to determine the number of cases and the attack rate [the population that is ill or meets the case definition divided by the population at risk]. The case definition allows investigators who are separated geographically to use the same criteria when evaluating the outbreak. The use of objective criteria in the case definition is critical to determining an accurate case number, as additional cases may be found and some cases may be excluded. This is especially true as the potential exists for panic and for subjective complaints to be confused with actual disease.

Once the attack rate has been determined, an outbreak can be described in terms of time, place, and person. These data will provide crucial information in determining the potential source of the outbreak. The epidemic curve is calculated based upon cases over time. In a point-source outbreak, which is most likely in a biological attack or terrorism situation, individuals are exposed to the disease agent in a fairly short time frame. The early phase of the epidemic curve may be compressed compared to a natural disease outbreak. In addition, the incubation period could be shorter than for a natural outbreak if individuals are exposed to higher inocula of the bioagent than would occur in the natural setting. The peak may occur in days or even hours. Later phases of the curve may also help determine if the disease is able to spread from person to person. Determining whether the disease is contagious will be extremely important for determining effective disease control measures. If the agent(s) is released at multiple times or sites, additional cases and multiple sequential peaks in the epidemic curve may also occur, something that happened with the mailed anthrax letters.

Once the disease is recognized, appropriate prophylaxis, treatment, and other measures to decrease disease spread, such as isolation (if needed for a contagious illness) would be instituted. The ultimate test of whether control measures are effective is determined by observation to see if they reduce ongoing illness or spread of disease.

In summary, it is important to understand that the recognition of and preparation for a biological attack will be similar to that for any infectious disease outbreak, but the surveillance, response, and other demands on resources will likely be of an unparalleled intensity. Public anxiety will be greater after an intentionally caused event; therefore, a sound risk-communication plan that involves public health authorities will be vital to an effective response and to allay the fears of the public. A strong public-health infrastructure with an effective epidemiological investigation capability, practical training programs, and preparedness plans are essential to prevent and control disease outbreaks, whether they are naturally occurring or intentional.

TABLE 1. Epidemiologic Clues of a BW or Bioterrorist Attack

The presence of a large outbreak with a similar disease or syndrome, especially in a discrete population
Many cases of unexplained diseases or deaths
More severe disease than is usually expected for a specific pathogen or failure to respond to standard therapy
Unusual routes of exposure for a pathogen, such as the inhalational route for diseases that normally occur through other exposures
A disease case or cases that are unusual for a given geographic area or transmission season
Disease normally transmitted by a vector that is not present in the local area
Multiple simultaneous or serial epidemics of different diseases in the same population
A single case of disease caused by an uncommon agent (smallpox, some viral hemorrhagic fevers, inhalational anthrax, pneumonic plague)
A disease that is unusual for an age group
Unusual strains or variants of organisms or antimicrobial resistance patterns different from those known to be circulating
A similar or exact genetic type among agents isolated from distinct sources at different times or locations
Higher attack rates among those exposed in certain areas, such as inside a building if released indoors, or lower rates in those inside a sealed building if released outside
Outbreaks of the same disease occurring simultaneously in noncontiguous areas
Zoonotic disease outbreaks
A zoonotic disease occurring in humans, but not animals
Intelligence of a potential attack, claims by a terrorist or aggressor of a release, and discovery of munitions, tampering, or other potential vehicle of spread (spray device, contaminated letter)

THE USE OF SYNDROMIC SURVEILLANCE IN A BIOLOGICAL ATTACK

The need to rapidly detect an intentionally caused disease outbreak has prompted a search for faster and more reliable methods for disease surveillance. "Syndromic surveillance" typically refers to the automated analysis of routinely collected health data that are available even before specific diagnoses are made. The rapid expansion of such surveillance systems in recent years can be attributed to 1) increasingly available and timely electronic data entered into accessible databases, 2) advances in informatics and statistics for data extraction, normalization, and detection of aberrations in temporal or spatial data, and 3) growing concerns about the threat of epidemics, influenza pandemics, bioterrorism and biowarfare. In many situations, syndromic surveillance systems may not detect outbreaks faster than traditional epidemiological surveillance methods. However, these systems may be able to provide information that can assist with the outbreak investigation, situational awareness, tracing the spread of outbreaks and the effectiveness of countermeasures.

Data that arise from an interaction with the health care system, but do not include confirmed or definitive diagnoses, can include early, non-specific diagnoses, such as "gastroenteritis," or procedures from initial encounters, such as "stool culture." They can be recorded as text in an electronic record, or through codes such as the International Classification of Diseases (ICD) or Current Procedural Terminology (CPT). A chief complaint such as "cough" can be entered in an Emergency Department electronic medical record, or "rash, unknown etiology" entered in a billing database. These data can also include initial impressions from emergency medical personnel on ambulance runs or calls to nurse advice lines or doctor's offices for information. Pre-encounter information obtained about the health of a population before presentation to a health care provider includes over-the-counter pharmacy sales for items such as cough syrup or anti-diarrheal medication. Behavioral changes can be detected in school or work absenteeism rates or internet queries. In general, the closer the data source is to a medical encounter (chief complaints, provider initial impressions, laboratory test orders), the more reliable the information.

To be analyzed for anomalies and compared to expected illness rates, indicator health events must be grouped into syndromes. Most data types, including pharmacy sales and prescriptions, laboratory tests, ambulance runs, chief complaints and diagnostic codes can be grouped into syndromes. Common syndrome groups include respiratory, gastrointestinal, rash, neurological, and febrile illnesses. A syndrome grouping schema based on ICD-9 codes, with an emphasis on bioterrorism detection, is available (www.bt.cdc.gov).

The most commonly promoted use of syndromic surveillance in a bioterrorism or biological warfare context is for early detection of an attack. Timely awareness of an increase in disease incidence can assist in mobilizing resources and potentially decrease associated morbidity and mortality. There are many examples of retrospective studies showing that syndromic surveillance can provide early warning of large community-wide disease outbreaks when compared to traditional disease reporting. Furthermore, it is assumed that such an alert could effect earlier etiologic diagnoses, and early institution of preventive measures such as vaccination and antibiotic prophylaxis, as well as prioritization of these measures to affected communities in time to reduce morbidity and mortality.

The characteristics of an outbreak that make it most likely to be detected by syndromic surveillance are 1) narrow distribution of the incubation period, 2) longer prodrome, 3) absence of a pathognomonic clinical sign that would speed diagnosis, and 4) diagnosis that is dependent on the use of specialized tests that are unlikely to be ordered. Not all biowarfare or terrorism-caused outbreaks will have these characteristics. In addition, early detection may or may not assist with determining whether the outbreak is the result of an intentional biological attack or not. Any disease outbreak must be investigated by appropriate public health officials, and law enforcement will only be involved if evidence arises that points to illegal activity. Early detection alone does not ensure recognition of a biological attack, but data in a syndromic system may help find clues that suggest an intentional event.

Besides early detection, syndromic surveillance systems can assist with the evaluation of the effectiveness of countermeasures, and provide support to epidemiological investigations by finding potential cases that have recently presented and have the same syndromic presentation as those already identified. It can also be used for situational awareness – providing reassurance during periods of high concern such as large public events or when bio-agents have been used on a small scale, such as the anthrax letter attacks, or after the potential ricin exposure in North London. With the use of environmental sensors for bioterrorism detection in large metropolitan areas, potential alerts can be shared with public health officials who can then carefully monitor syndromic data in the same geographic area.

TEN STEPS IN THE MANAGEMENT OF POTENTIAL BIOLOGICAL CASUALTIES

Military medical personnel will require a firm understanding of certain key elements of biological defense to manage effectively the consequences of a biological attack amidst the confusion expected on the modern battlefield. Civilian providers who might be called upon to respond to a bioterrorist attack require a similar understanding. Familiarity with the characteristics, pathogenesis, modes of transmission, diagnostic modalities, and available treatment options for each of the potential agents thus becomes imperative. Acquiring such an understanding is relatively straightforward once the identity of the agent is known; many references (e.g., Army FM 8-284, NATO AMedP-6), including this handbook, exist to assist medical personnel in agent-specific therapy. A larger problem presents itself when the identity of a causative agent is unknown. In some cases, an attack may be threatened, but it may remain unclear as to whether such an attack has actually occurred. Similarly, it may be initially unclear whether casualties are due to the intentional release of a biological agent or a chemical agent, or whether they are due to a naturally occurring infectious disease outbreak, an emerging infectious disease, an accidental toxic industrial exposure, or even mass psychogenic illness. We recommend here a ten-step process to guide medical personnel in the evaluation and management of intentional outbreaks of unknown origin and etiology. We feel that such an algorithmic approach (as exemplified by the Advanced Trauma Life Support Course (ATLS) sponsored by the American College of Surgeons) is desirable when dealing with the unknown, especially under the austere conditions and chaos expected on the modern battlefield.

1. Maintain an index of suspicion. In the case of chemical or conventional warfare and terrorism, the sinister nature of an attack might be obvious. Victims would likely succumb in close temporal and geographic proximity to a dispersal or explosive device (i.e., clustered in time and space). Complicating discovery of the sinister nature of a biological attack, however, is the fact that bio-agents possess inherent incubation periods. These incubation periods, typically days to even weeks in length, permit the wide dispersion of victims (in both time and space). Moreover, they make it likely that the 'first responder' to a biological attack would not be the traditional first responder (fire, police, and paramedical personnel), but rather medics, primary care physicians, emergency room personnel, and public health officials. In such circumstances, the maintenance of a healthy 'index of suspicion' by a medical provider is imperative if a timely diagnosis is to be made and prompt therapy instituted.

Additionally, with many of the diseases typically regarded as potential weapons, very early intervention is mandatory if a good patient outcome is to be achieved. Anthrax, botulism, plague, and smallpox are readily prevented if patients are provided proper antibiotics, antisera, and/or vaccination promptly after exposure. Conversely, all of these diseases may prove fatal if therapy or prophylaxis is delayed until classic symptoms develop. Unfortunately, symptoms in the early, or prodromal, phase of these illnesses are non-specific, making diagnosis difficult. Moreover, many weaponizable bioagent infections, such as brucellosis, Q fever, and Venezuelan equine encephalitis (VEE), may present simply as undifferentiated febrile illnesses. Without a high index of suspicion, it is unlikely that medical personnel, especially at lower echelons of care, removed from sophisticated laboratory and preventive medicine resources, will promptly arrive at a proper diagnosis and institute appropriate therapy.

II. Protect yourself. Before medical personnel approach a potential biological casualty, they must first take steps to protect themselves. These steps may involve a combination of physical, chemical, and immunologic forms of protection. On the battlefield, physical protection typically consists of a protective mask. Designed primarily with chemical vapor hazards in mind, the M-40 series mask certainly provides adequate protection against all aerosolized bioagent threats. In fact, a HEPA-filter (or even a simple surgical) mask will often afford adequate protection against all bio-agents, although not against chemical threats. Chemical protection refers, in general, to the pre- and/or postexposure administration of antibiotics; such strategies are discussed on an agent-specific basis elsewhere in this book. Immunologic protection principally involves active vaccination and, at present time, applies mainly to protection against anthrax and smallpox. Again, specific vaccination strategies are discussed throughout this book. Obviously, not all of these protective strategies would be applicable in every situation.

III. Assess the patient. This initial assessment is somewhat analogous to the primary survey of ATLS management. As such, before attention is given to specific management, airway adequacy should be assessed and breathing and circulation problems addressed. The initial assessment is conducted before decontamination is accomplished and thus should be brief, but the need for decontamination and for the administration of antidotes for rapid-acting chemical agents (nerve agents and cyanide) should be determined at this time. Historical information of potential interest to the clinician should also be gathered, and might include information about illnesses among other unit members, the presence of unusual munitions, food and water procurement sources, vector exposure, vaccination history, travel history, occupational duties, and MOPP status. Physical exam at this point should concentrate on the pulmonary and neuromuscular systems, as well as any unusual rashes or bleeding.

IV. Decontaminate as appropriate. Decontamination plays a very important role in the approach to chemical casualty management. The incubation period of bio-agents, however, makes it unlikely that victims of a biological attack will present for medical care until days after exposure. At this point, the need for decontamination is likely minimal or non-existent. In those rare cases where decontamination is warranted, simple soap and water bathing will usually suffice. Certainly, standard military decontamination solutions (such as hypochlorite), typically employed in cases of chemical agent contamination, will be effective against all bio-agents. In fact, even 0.1% bleach reliably kills anthrax spores, the hardiest of bio-agents. Routine use of caustic substances, especially on human skin, however, is rarely warranted after a biological attack. More information on decontamination is included elsewhere in this text. It must also be kept in mind that a biological attack constitutes a criminal act and that hasty ill-considered decontamination risks destroying valuable evidence.

V. Establish a diagnosis. With decontamination (where warranted) accomplished, a more thorough attempt to establish a diagnosis can be carried out. This attempt, somewhat analogous to the secondary survey used in the ATLS approach, should involve a combination of clinical, epidemiological, and laboratory examinations. The amount of expertise and support available to the clinician will vary at each echelon of care. At higher echelons, a full range of laboratory capabilities might enable prompt definitive diagnoses. At lower echelons, every attempt should be made to obtain diagnostic specimens from representative patients and forward these

TABLE 1. Diagnostic Matrix: Chemical & Biological Casualties

	Rapid Onset	Delayed Onset
Respiratory	Nerve Agents Cyanide Mustard Lewisite Phosgene SEB Inhalation	Inhalational Anthrax Pneumonic Plague Pneumonic Tularemia Q Fever SEB Inhalation Ricin Inhalation Mustard Lewisite Phosgene
Neurological	Nerve Agents Cyanide	Botulism-Peripheral Symptoms VEE-CNS Symptoms

through laboratory channels. Nasal swabs (important for culture and polymerase chain reaction (PCR), even if the clinician is unsure *which* organisms are present), blood cultures, serum, sputum cultures, blood and urine for toxin analysis, throat swabs, should be obtained. Environmental samples should also be collected according to established protocols, and analyzed accordingly. In no case, however, should the performance of (or unavailability of) laboratory studies delay empiric diagnosis and therapy.

While awaiting laboratory confirmation, a physician should attempt to make a presumptive (empiric) diagnosis. Access (at higher echelons of care) to infectious disease, preventive medicine, and other specialists, can assist in this process. At lower echelons, the clinician should, at the very least, be familiar with the concept of syndromic diagnosis. Chemical and biowarfare diseases can be generally divided into those that present "immediately" with little or no incubation period (principally the chemical agents) and those with a considerable delay in presentation (principally the bioagents). Moreover, biowarfare diseases are likely to present as one of a limited number of clinical syndromes. Plague, tularemia, and staphylococcal enterotoxin (SEB) disease all may present as pneumonia. Botulism and Venezuelan equine encephalitis (VEE) may present with peripheral and central neuromuscular findings, respectively. This allows for the construction of a simple diagnostic matrix as shown in Table 1. Even syndromic diagnosis, however, is complicated by the fact that many biowarfare diseases (VEE, Q fever, brucellosis) may present simply as undifferentiated febrile illnesses and remain that way throughout their course. Moreover, other diseases (anthrax, plague, tularemia, smallpox) present undifferentiated febrile prodromes, but exhibit characteristic signs and symptoms in due course.

VI. Render prompt treatment. Unfortunately, it is precisely in the prodromal phase of many diseases that therapy is most likely to be effective. For this reason, empiric therapy of pneumonia or undifferentiated febrile illness on the battlefield or in a potential bioterrorism scenario might be indicated under certain circumstances. Table 2 was constructed by eliminating from consideration those diseases for which definitive therapy is not warranted, not available, or not essential. Those that remain, therefore, have some specific (as opposed to merely supportive) therapy available. Empiric treatment of respiratory casualties (patients with undifferentiated febrile illnesses who might have prodromal anthrax, plague, or tularemia would all be managed similarly) might then be entertained. Doxycycline, for example, is effective against most strains of *Bacillus anthracis*, *Yersinia pestis*, and *Francisella tularensis*, as well as against *Coxiella burnetii*, and the *Brucellae*. Other tetracyclines and fluoroquinolones might also be considered. Similarly, rapid-onset respiratory casualties might be treated empirically using a cyanide antidote kit, while rapid-onset neurological casualties might warrant prompt empiric therapy with a Nerve Agent Antidote Kit. Keep in mind that such therapy is, in no way, a substitute for a careful and thorough diagnostic evaluation, when conditions permit such an evaluation.

TABLE 2. CW & BW Diseases Potentially Benefitting From Prompt Specific Empiric Therapy

	Rapid Onset	Delayed Onset
Respiratory	Nerve Agents Cyanide	Inhalational Anthrax Pneumonic Plague Pneumonic Tularemia
Neurological	Nerve Agents	Botulism

VII. Practice good infection control. Standard precautions provide adequate protection against most infectious diseases, including most of those potentially employed in a biological attack. Anthrax, tularemia, brucellosis, glanders, Q fever, VEE, and the toxin-mediated diseases are not generally contagious, and victims can be safely managed using standard precautions. Such precautions should be familiar to all clinicians. Under certain circumstances, however, one of three forms of transmission-based precautions would be warranted. Smallpox victims should, wherever possible, be managed using 'airborne precautions' (including, ideally, a HEPA-filter mask). Pneumonic plague warrants the use of 'droplet precautions' (which include, among other measures, the wearing of a simple surgical mask), and certain viral hemorrhagic fevers and smallpox require 'contact precautions.'

VIII. Alert the proper authorities. In any military context, the command should immediately be notified of casualties potentially exposed to chemical or bio-agents. The clinical laboratory receiving specimens should also be notified. This will enable laboratory personnel to take proper precautions when handling them and will also permit the optimal use of various diagnostic modalities. Chemical Corps and preventive medicine personnel should be contacted to assist in the delineation of contaminated areas and the search for additional victims.

In a civilian context, such notification would typically be made through local and/or regional health department channels. In the U.S., larger cities often have their own health departments. In most other areas, the county represents the lowest echelon health jurisdiction. In some rural areas, practitioners would access the state health department directly. Once alerted, local and regional health authorities are normally well-versed on the mechanisms for requesting additional support from health officials at higher jurisdictions. Each practitioner should have a point of contact with such agencies and should be familiar with mechanisms for contacting them before a crisis arises.

IX. Assist in the epidemiologic investigation and manage the psychological consequences. All healthcare providers should have a basic understanding of epidemiological principles. Even under austere conditions, a rudimentary outbreak investigation may assist in diagnosis and in the discovery of additional biowarfare victims. Clinicians should, at the very least, query patients about illness onset and symptoms, potential exposures, ill unit members, food/water sources, unusual munitions or spray devices, and vector exposures. Early discovery of additional cases through an expedient epidemiologic investigation might, in turn, permit postexposure prophylaxis (PEP), thereby avoiding excess morbidity and mortality. Public health officials would normally conduct more formal and thorough epidemiologic investigations and should be contacted as soon as one suspects the possibility of a biological attack. In a military setting, preventive medicine officers, field sanitation personnel, epidemiology technicians, environmental science officers, and veterinary officers are all available to assist the clinician in conducting an epidemiologic investigation.

In addition to implementing specific medical countermeasures and initiating an epidemiologic investigation, the clinician must be prepared to address the psychological effects of a known, suspected, or feared exposure. Such an exposure (or threat of exposure) can provoke fear and anxiety in the population, and may result in overwhelming numbers of patients seeking medical evaluation. Many of these will likely have unexplained symptoms and many may demand antidotes and other therapies. Moreover, symptoms due to anxiety and autonomic arousal, as well as the side effects of postexposure antibiotic prophylaxis may suggest prodromal disease due to biological-agent exposure, and may pose challenges in differential diagnosis. This 'behavioral contagion' is best prevented by good, proactive, risk communication from health and governmental authorities to community leaders and the media. Such risk communication should include a realistic assessment of the risk of exposure, information about the resulting disease, steps to be taken, and points of contact for suspected exposure. Risk communication must be timely, accurate, consistent, and well-coordinated.

Effective risk communication is predicated upon the pre-existence of thorough risk communication plans and tactical approaches. Similarly, plans must be made to rapidly deploy resources for the initial evaluation and administration of postexposure prophylaxis (ideally decentralized to unit level on the battlefield or to residential areas in a civilian context). Finally, plans must be made to proactively develop patient and contact tracing and vaccine screening tools, to access stockpiled vaccines and medications, and to identify and prepare local facilities and healthcare teams for the care of mass casualties.

X. Maintain Proficiency and Spread the Word. Fortunately, the threats of biological warfare and bioterrorism have remained theoretical ones for most medical personnel. Inability to practice casualty management, however, leads to a rapid deterioration of skills and knowledge. It is imperative that the medic maintains proficiency in dealing with this low-probability, but high-consequence problem. This can be done, in part, by availing oneself of several resources. The USAMRIID (www.usamriid.army.mil) web site provides a wealth of information, including the full text of this handbook, as well as links to many other useful sites. Numerous satellite television broadcasts sponsored by USAMRIID, as well as other video course resources, provide in-depth discussion and training in medical biodefense. CD-ROM training aids are also available, and a field manual (Army FM 8-284) summarizes biowarfare disease management recommendations. Finally, medical personnel, once aware of the threat and trained to deal with it, must ensure that other personnel in their units receive training as well. It is only through ongoing training that personnel will be ready to deal with the threat posed by biological weapons. By familiarizing yourself with the contents of this handbook, you have taken a large step towards such readiness.

BACTERIAL AGENTS

Bacteria are unicellular organisms that vary in shape and size from spherical cells (cocci) with a diameter of 0.5-1.0 μmm (micrometer), to long rod-shaped organisms (bacilli) which may be from 1-5 μmm. Chains of some bacilli may exceed 50 μmm in length. The shape of the bacterial cell is determined by the rigid cell wall. The interior of the cell contains the nuclear material (DNA), cytoplasm, and cell membrane; all are necessary for the life of the bacterium. Many bacteria also have glycoproteins on their outer surfaces which aid in bacterial attachment to cell-surface receptors. Under special circumstances, some types of bacteria (such as *Bacillus anthracis*) can transform into spores. The spore of the bacterial cell is more resistant to cold, heat, drying, chemicals, UV light, and radiation than the vegetative bacterium itself. Spores are a dormant form of the bacterium and, like the seeds of plants, they can germinate when conditions are favorable. Aerosolized spores that are 1-5 μmm in size may be inhaled deeply into the terminal bronchioles and alveoli of the lungs of humans and animals.

The term rickettsia generally applies to very small, gram-negative coccobacilli of the genera *Rickettsia* and *Coxiella*. Rickettsiae are distinct from classical bacteria in their inability to grow (with rare exceptions) in the absence of a living eukaryotic host cell (typically endothelial cells). Like the classical bacteria, however, rickettsiae are susceptible to treatment with antibiotics.

Bacteria generally cause disease in human beings and animals by one of two mechanisms: by invading host tissues, and/or by producing poisons (toxins). Many pathogenic bacteria utilize both mechanisms. The diseases they produce often respond to specific therapy with antibiotics. It is important to distinguish between the disease-causing organism and the name of the disease it causes (in parentheses below). This manual covers several of the bacteria or rickettsiae considered to be potential threat bioagents: *Bacillus anthracis* (anthrax), *Brucella* spp. (brucellosis), *Burkholderia mallei* (glanders), *Burholderia pseudomallei* (melioidosis), *Yersinia pestis* (plague), *Francisella tularensis* (tularemia), and *Coxiella burnetii* (Q fever).

Anthrax

SUMMARY

Signs and Symptoms of Inhalational Anthrax (IA): Incubation period is generally 1-6 d, although longer periods have been noted. Fever, malaise, fatigue, dry cough, and mild chest discomfort progress to severe respiratory distress with dyspnea, diaphoresis, stridor, cyanosis, and shock. Death typically occurs within 24-36 h after onset of severe symptoms.

Diagnosis: Physical findings are non-specific. A widened mediastinum and pleural effusions may be seen on CXR or CT scan in later stages of illness. The organism is detectable by Gram stain of the blood and by blood culture late in the course of illness.

Treatment: Although effectiveness may be limited after symptoms are present, high-dose IV antibiotic treatment with ciprofloxacin or doxycycline combined with one or two additional antibiotics are indicated. Intensive supportive therapy will be necessary.

Prophylaxis: An FDA-licensed vaccine is available. Vaccine schedule is 0.5 ml intramuscularly at 0 and 4 weeks, then 6, 12, and 18 months (primary series), followed by annual boosters for pre-event prophylaxis. For known or imminent exposure (postexposure prophylaxis), vaccine schedule is 0, 2 and 4 weeks subcutaneously in combination with oral ciprofloxacin or doxycycline for 60 days. The licensed vaccine schedule is then resumed at 6 months.

Isolation and Decontamination: Standard precautions for healthcare workers. Avoid invasive procedures or autopsy; but if performed, all instruments and proximate environment should be thoroughly disinfected with a sporicidal agent (e.g., hypochlorite).

OVERVIEW

Bacillus anthracis, the causative agent of anthrax, is a gram-positive, sporulating rod. The spores are the usual infective form. Naturally occurring anthrax is primarily a zoonotic disease of herbivores, with cattle, sheep, goats, and horses serving as the usual domesticated animal hosts, but other animals may be infected. Humans generally contract the disease when handling contaminated hair, wool, hides, flesh, blood, and excreta of infected animals and from manufactured products such as bone meal. Infection is introduced through scratches or abrasions of the skin, wounds, inhaling spores, eating insufficiently cooked infected meat, or by fly bites. The primary concern for intentional infection by this organism is through inhalation after aerosol dissemination of spores. All human populations are susceptible. The spores are very stable and may remain viable for many years in soil and water. They resist sunlight for varying periods.

HISTORY AND SIGNIFICANCE

Anthrax spores were weaponized by the U.S. in the 1950s and 1960s before the old U.S. offensive program was terminated. Other countries, including the Soviet Union and Iraq, have weaponized this agent and others were suspected of doing so. In the fall of 2001, anthrax spores were delivered in the U.S. mail, resulting in 22 cases of confirmed or suspected anthrax disease. Anthrax bacteria are easy to cultivate and spore production is readily induced. Moreover, the spores are highly resistant to sunlight, heat, and disinfectants - properties which create concerns for environmental persistence after an attack. This agent can be produced in either a wet or dried form, stabilized for weaponization by an adversary, and delivered as an aerosol cloud either from a line source (such as an aircraft flying upwind of friendly positions), or as a point source (from a spray device). Theoretically, coverage of a large ground area could also be accomplished by multiple spray bomblets disseminated from a missile warhead at a predetermined height above the ground.

CLINICAL FEATURES

Anthrax presents as three distinct clinical syndromes in humans: cutaneous, gastrointestinal, and inhalational disease.

Cutaneous anthrax. The cutaneous form (also referred to as "malignant pustule") is the most common naturally occurring form of anthrax. It occurs most frequently on the hands and forearms of persons working with infected livestock or livestock products, but during epizootics it has been transmitted to humans by the bites of flies, and more recently occurred in as many as 11 people exposed to anthrax spores in the U.S. mail. After a 1 to 12 day (mean 7 day) incubation period, a painless or pruritic papule forms at the site of exposure, enlarging into a round ulcer by the next day. Vesicles or bullae containing clear or serosanguinous fluid and bacilli may form on the edge of the ulcer, which can be surrounded by various degrees of non-pitting edema. The ulcer subsequently dries and forms a coal-black scab (eschar), which falls off over the ensuing 1 to 2 weeks. Regional lymphadenopathy with associated systemic symptoms can occur. If untreated, this local infection may disseminate into a fatal systemic infection in 10-20% of cases. Treated, mortality is less than 1 %.

Gastrointestinal (GI) anthrax is rare in humans, and is contracted by eating insufficiently cooked meat from infected animals. Infection is thought to occur as a result of the ingestion of viable vegetative organisms in contrast to spores. The two forms of GI anthrax, oropharyngeal and intestinal, have incubation periods of 1-6 days. Disease in **oropharyngeal** anthrax is heralded by the onset of fever and severe pharyngitis, followed by oral ulcers which progress from whitish patches to tan or gray pseudomembranes (often over a palatine tonsil and unilateral, but variable in location). Other signs and symptoms include dysphagia, regional lymphadenopathy (non-purulent), and severe neck swelling (often unilateral). Edema can lead to airway compromise, and disease can progress to sepsis, with case fatality rates (CFR) of 10 to 50%. **Intestinal** anthrax begins with fever, nausea, vomiting, and focal abdominal pain. These symptoms can progress to hematemesis, hematochezia or melena, massive serosanguinous or hemorrhagic ascites, and sepsis. Overall CFR is greater than 50%. Some evidence exists for a mild, self-limited gastroenteritis syndrome associated with intestinal anthrax, but this is poorly described.

Inhalational (IA) anthrax. Endemic inhalational anthrax, known as Woolsorters' disease, is also an extremely rare infection contracted by inhaling the spores. It has historically occurred in an industrial setting, mainly among workers who handle infected hides, wool, and furs. Because of the rarity of human IA, a single case of this disease should be presumed to be as a result of intentional exposure to anthrax until proved otherwise. After an incubation period of 1 to 6 days,* a non-specific febrile syndrome begins. Fever, malaise, headache, fatigue, and drenching sweats are often present, sometimes in association with nausea, vomiting, confusion, a nonproductive cough, and mild chest discomfort. Physical findings are typically non-specific in the early phase of the disease. Patients are often tachycardic, and despite normal lung physical exams, often have (albeit

*During an outbreak of IA in the Soviet Union in 1979, persons are reported to have become ill up to 6 weeks after an aerosol release occurred. Studies performed in nonhuman primates demonstrate that anthrax spores remain in the lung for up to 100 days.

sometimes subtle at this stage) evidence of mediastinal widening (hemorrhagic mediastinitis) or pleural effusions on CXR or CT scan. These initial symptoms generally last 2-5 days and can be followed by a short period of apparent improvement (hours to 2-3 days), culminating in the abrupt development of severe respiratory distress with dyspnea, diaphoresis, stridor, and cyanosis. Septicemia, shock, and death usually follow within 24-36 h after the onset of respiratory distress unless dramatic life-saving efforts are initiated. Historically, IA has been complicated by hemorrhagic meningitis in up to 50% of cases and GI hemorrhage in 80% of cases. For the attacks of 2001, CFR was only 45%, while before this time CFRs for IA were > 85%. This better outcome was likely a reflection of advancements in intensive care medicine and the aggressive treatment of recent victims.

DIAGNOSIS

All forms of anthrax disease are diagnosed using a combination of clinical and laboratory findings.

Cutaneous anthrax. The key to diagnosis centers upon the presence of the characteristic painless skin lesion which progresses to a vesicle, ulcer, then eschar, with surrounding edema. While arachnid bites or cutaneous tularemia may appear similar, these lesions are characteristically painful. Known exposure history or risk factors may also be present. To perform Gram stain and bacterial culture of the lesion, samples should be collected by using two dry Dacron or rayon swabs, ideally with the fluid of an unopened vesicle. If no vesicle is present, apply moistened swabs (sterile saline) to an eschar or in the base of an ulcer. Gram stain often demonstrates large gram-positive bacilli if the patient has not yet received antibiotics. If the Gram stain and culture are negative, collect a 4-mm punch biopsy (or two if both eschar and vesicle are present) of the leading margin of the lesion for general histology and immunostaining. Blood culture should be performed in all patients suspected of having anthrax.

Gastrointestinal anthrax. History of exposure to or ingestion of the meat of sick animals should be elicited. Clinical suspicion should be elevated for multiple cases of similar disease. **Oropharyngeal** disease can mimic diphtheria, and vaccination and travel history should be queried. Gram stain and culture of the oral lesion may be positive for *B. anthracis* if collected before initiation of antibiotics. **Intestinal** anthrax may mimic acute gastroenteritis, acute abdomen with peritonitis (thus focal and rebound tenderness), or dysentery.

Abdominal radiographic studies are non-specific, sometimes showing diffuse air-fluid levels, bowel thickening, and peritoneal fluid. Surgical findings may include hemorrhagic mesenteric adenitis, serosanguinous to hemorrhagic ascites, bowel ulceration (usually ileum and cecum), edema, and necrosis. Stool culture is sometimes positive in intestinal anthrax. Peritoneal fluid should be sent for Gram stain, culture, immunostaining, and PCR. Blood should be collected for culture, serology (paired frozen sera 3-4 weeks apart, -70°C) and PCR (lavender tube, refrigerated) in patients with either form of GI disease. Ascitic fluid can be sent for culture, PCR, and immunostaining.

Inhalational anthrax. Early IA is a non-specific syndrome which may be difficult to distinguish clinically from other illnesses. Notably absent in IA are upper respiratory symptoms (rhinorrhea, coryza, congestion) as one would see with influenza. Pneumonia generally does not occur; therefore, lung exam may be unrevealing and organisms are not typically seen in the sputum. Patients suspected of having IA should have a complete blood count (CBC), blood culture, and serum electrolytes. White blood cell count is typically elevated only slightly at presentation (mean 9,800/microliter in the 2001 cases) with a neutrophil predominance. Hemoconcentration may be evidenced by elevated serum sodium and hematocrit. Mildly elevated serum aspartate aminotransferase (AST) and alanine aminotransferase (ALT) may be present as well as hypoalbuminemia. *B. anthracis* will be detectable even in the early phase of disease by routine blood culture and may even be seen on Gram stain of blood later in the course of the illness; however, even one or two doses of antibiotics will render blood (and other sites) sterile. In patients with neurologic symptoms, cerebrospinal fluid (CSF) may show evidence of hemorrhagic meningitis with numerous gram-positive bacilli. Pleural effusions may be large and bloody; Gram stain may show organisms. If cultures are sterile, blood and other fluids may be sent for PCR; CSF, pleural fluid, and tissue may be sent for immunostaining; and acute and convalescent serum may be collected for serology. All patients suspected of having IA should have a CXR to look for mediastinal adenitis (seen as a widened mediastinum or mediastinal "fullness") and pleural effusions. If normal, a chest CT scan should be performed. In the attacks of 2001, CXR and/or chest CT were abnormal in all cases.

MEDICAL MANAGEMENT

Inhalational anthrax. Early initiation of appropriate antibiotics is paramount for patient survival of IA. Initial therapy for adults with IA due to a strain with unknown antibiotic susceptibilities should include ciprofloxacin (400 mg iv q 12 h for adults, and 10-15 mg/kg intravenously q12 h (up to 1 g/day) for children) OR doxycycline (200 mg intravenous load, followed by 100 mg intravenous q12 h for adults and children > 8 yr and >45 kg, and 2.2mg/kg q12 h for children < 8 yr (up to 200 mg/days))* PLUS one or two additional antibiotics effective against anthrax. Some additional antibiotics to which naturally occurring strains of *B. anthracis* are susceptible include imipenem, meropenem, daptomycin, quinupristin-dalfopristin, linezolid, vancomycin, rifampin, macrolides (e.g., erythromycin, azithromycin, and clarithromycin), clindamycin, chloramphenocol, and aminoglycosides (e.g., gentamicin). While optimal combination antibiotic therapy for IA is not known, many infectious disease physicians have suggested a combination of a quinolone, clindamycin, and rifampin for susceptible *B. anthracis* strains. Penicillin (or other beta-lactam antibiotics) should NEVER be used as monotherapy for severe anthrax disease as the *B. anthracis* genome encodes for both constitutive and inducible beta-lactamases and resistance may occur in vivo despite apparent in vitro susceptibility. Antibiotic choices must be adjusted for strain susceptibility patterns, and consultation with an infectious disease physician is imperative. If meningitis is suspected, at least one antibiotic with good cerebrospinal fluid (CSF) penetration (e.g., rifampin or chloramphenicol) should be used, as quinolones and tetracyclines do not enter the CSF well. Generally, ciprofloxacin or doxycycline use is avoided during pregnancy and in children due to safety concerns; however, a consensus group and the American Academy of Pediatrics have suggested that they should still be used as first line therapy in life-threatening anthrax disease until strain susceptibilities are known. In fact, ciprofloxacin has been approved by the FDA for prophylaxis and treatment of anthrax in children. Recommended treatment duration is at least 60 days, and should be changed to oral therapy as clinical condition improves.

In the event of a mass-casualty situation intravenous antibiotics may not be available. In this case oral ciprofloxacin OR doxycycline may have to suffice as initial therapy. The doses for ciprofloxacin are 500 mg PO bid for adults, and 10-15 mg/kg PO bid (up to 1 g/day) for children. The doses for doxycycline are 200 mg PO initially then 100 mg PO bid thereafter for

*Other quinolone antibiotics (levofloxacin, trovofloxacin) or tetracyclines (minocycline, tetracycline) would likely be affective as well, although they have not been specifically approved by the FDA for this purpose.

adults (or children > 8 yr and > 45 kg), and 2.2 mg/kg PO bid (up to 200 mg/day) for children < 8 yr.

Supportive therapy for shock, fluid volume deficit, and adequacy of airway may be needed. In the IA cases from the 2001 attacks, aggressive drainage of pleural effusions seemed to improve clinical outcome. Corticosteroids may be considered as adjunct therapy in patients with severe edema or meningitis, based upon experience in treating other bacterial diseases. Human anthrax immune globulin can be obtained as a therapy for IA under an IND from the CDC (see **Appendix L** for instructions on INDs).

Cutaneous anthrax. Uncomplicated cutaneous anthrax disease should be treated initially with either ciprofloxacin (500 mg PO bid for adults or 10-15 mg/kg/d divided bid (up to 1000 mg/d) for children) or doxycycline (100 mg PO bid for adults, 5 mg/kg/d divided bid for children less than 8 yr (up to 200 mg/d)). If the strain proves to be penicillin susceptible, then the treatment may be switched to amoxicillin (500 mg PO tid for adults or 80 mg/kg PO divided tid (up to 1500 mg/d) for children). While the *B. anthracis* genome encodes for beta-lactamases, the organism may still respond to penicillins (such as amoxicillin) if slowly growing as in localized cutaneous disease. In the event that the exposure route is unknown or suspected to be intentional, then antibiotics should be continued for at least 60 d. If the exposure is known to have been due to contact with infected livestock or their products, then 7-10 days of antibiotics may suffice. For patients with significant edema, non-steroidal anti-inflammatory drugs (NSAIDS) or corticosteroids may be of benefit. Debridement of lesions is not indicated. If systemic illness accompanies cutaneous anthrax, then intravenous antibiotics should be administered as per the inhalational anthrax recommendations discussed above.

Gastrointestinal anthrax. Documentation of clinical experience in treating oropharyngeal and intestinal anthrax is limited. Supportive care to include fluid, shock, and airway management should be anticipated. Both forms of GI disease should receive the intravenous antibiotic regimen described for inhalational anthrax above. For oropharyngeal anthrax, airway compromise is a significant risk, and consideration should be given for the early administration of corticosteroids to reduce the development of airway edema. If despite medical therapy, airway compromise develops, early airway control with intubation should be considered. Incision and drainage of affected lymph nodes is not generally indicated. No specific guidance exists for drainage of ascites in patients with intestinal anthrax. However, large fluid collections could at a minimum compromise respiration and consideration should be given to therapeutic (and potentially diagnostic) paracentesis.

Infection Control. Standard precautions are recommended for patient care in all forms of anthrax disease. There are no data to suggest direct person-to-person spread from any form of anthrax disease. However, for patients with systemic anthrax disease, especially before antibiotic initiation, invasive procedures, autopsy, or embalming of remains could potentially lead to the generation of infectious droplets; thus, such procedures should be avoided when possible. After an invasive procedure or autopsy, the instruments and materials used should be autoclaved or incinerated, and the immediate environment where the procedure took place should be thoroughly disinfected with a sporicidal agent. Iodine can be used, but must be used at disinfectant strengths, as antiseptic-strength iodophors are not usually sporicidal. Chlorine, in the form of sodium or calcium hypochlorite, can also be used, but with the caution that the activity of hypochlorites is greatly reduced in the presence of organic material.

The clinical laboratory should be warned before the delivery of suspected anthrax specimens as growth of *B. anthracis* in culture requires biosafety level (BSL)-2 precautions.

Animal anthrax experience indicates that incineration of carcasses and sterilization of contaminated ground is the environmental control method of choice. A prior recommendation was deep burial (at least 6 feet deep) in pits copiously lined with lye (sodium hydroxide); however, this practice may still leave a significant proportion of viable spores. This has led a consensus group to recommend "serious consideration" of cremation of human anthrax victim remains.

PROPHYLAXIS

Vaccine: A licensed vaccine *Biothrax®* (Anthrax Vaccine Adsorbed (AVA) Emergent Biosolutions, Rockville, MD) is derived from sterile culture fluid supernatant taken from an attenuated (non-encapsulated) strain of anthrax. Therefore, this vaccine does not contain live or dead organisms. The licensed vaccination series consists of five 0.5-ml intramuscular total doses: one each at 0 and 4 wks; then 6, 12, and 18 mos, followed by yearly boosters. Current Department of Defense (DoD) policy for missed doses (for those individuals required to remain immune) is to administer the missed dose ASAP and reset the timeline for the series based upon the most recent dose. On December 15, 2005, the FDA issued a Final Rule & Order on the license status of AVA. After reviewing extensive scientific evidence and carefully considering comments from the public, the FDA again determined that AVA is licensed for the prevention of anthrax, regardless of the route of exposure. AVA is licensed only for pre-exposure prophylaxis of anthrax in adults (ages >18 and < 65). It is available for pre-exposure use in children, and postexposure prophylaxis (PEP –administered subcutaneously) in adults and children only under an Investigational New Drug (IND) protocol or an Emergency Use Authorization (EUA) through the CDC and DoD. As with all vaccines, the degree of protection depends upon the magnitude of the challenge dose; vaccine-induced protection could presumably be overwhelmed by extremely high spore challenge. Thus, even fully vaccinated personnel should receive antibiotic prophylaxis if exposed to aerosolized anthrax, per the guidelines given below.

Contraindications for use of AVA include hypersensitivity reaction to a previous dose of vaccine and age < 18 or > 65. Reasons for temporary deferment of the vaccine include pregnancy, active infection with fever, or a course of immune-suppressing drugs such as steroids. Reactogenicity is mild to moderate. Up to 30% of recipients may experience mild discomfort at the inoculation site for up to 72 h (e.g., tenderness, erythema, edema, pruritus), fewer experience moderate reactions, while less than 1% may experience more severe local reactions, potentially limiting use of the arm for 1-2 days. Modest systemic reactions (e.g., myalgia, malaise, low-grade fever) are uncommon, and severe systemic reactions such as anaphylaxis, which precludes additional vaccination, are rare. The vaccine should be stored between 2-6°C (refrigerator temperature, not frozen).

Current DoD policy is to require AVA vaccination for active-duty personnel (without specific contraindications) as well as some emergency-essential DoD civilians and contractors, who deploy for more than 15 consecutive d or more than 15 cumulative d over 12 mos, to designated "higher-threat" areas. The vaccination series should be initiated, when feasible, at least 45 d before deployment. Details of the DoD (and service-specific guidance) can be found at: http://www.anthrax.osd.mil/resource/policies/policies.asp.

AVA is recommended for persons who handle high concentrations of spores and potentially infected animals and those who work in spore-contaminated areas.

AVA has been included in the Strategic National Stockpile (SNS) for PEP use in the event of a biological attack, under either an IND protocol or an EUA.

Antibiotics: No antibiotics are approved for pre-exposure prophylaxis of anthrax. Thus, official DoD policy is not to initiate prophylactic antibiotics until AFTER an attack is suspected to have occurred. After a suspected exposure to aerosolized anthrax of unknown antibiotic susceptibility, prophylaxis with ciprofloxacin (500 mg PO bid for adults, and 10-15 mg/kg PO bid (up to 1 g/day) for children) OR doxycycline (100 mg PO bid for adults or children >8 yr and >45 kg, and 2.2 mg/kg PO bid (up to 200 mg/day) for children < 8yr) should be initiated immediately. Should an attack be confirmed as anthrax, antibiotics should be continued for variable lengths of time dependent upon the patient's vaccination status. If antibiotic susceptibilities allow, patients who cannot tolerate tetracyclines or quinolones can be switched to amoxicillin (500 mg PO tid for adults and 80 mg/kg divided tid (1.5 g/day) in children). AVA is a critical part of postexposure prophylaxis for inhaled anthrax; without vaccine, victims exposed to inhaled anthrax spores are unlikely to develop the immunity necessary to prevent disease caused by spores that germinate after antibiotics are discontinued. The Advisory Committee on Immunization Practices (ACIP) recommends a postexposure regimen of 60 days of appropriate antimicrobial prophylaxis combined with three doses (0, 2, and 4 weeks) for previously unvaccinated persons aged >18 yrs. The licensed vaccination schedule can be resumed at 6 mos. The first dose of vaccine should be administered within 10 days, Persons for whom vaccination has been delayed should extend antimicrobial use to 14 days after the third dose (even if this practice might result in use of antimicrobials for > 60 d. (*MMWR* 59(RR-6):1-30.2010) Patients who were either partially* or fully vaccinated** before the attack should continue with the licensed vaccination schedule and take antibiotics for at least 60 days. Upon discontinuation of antibiotics, patients should be closely observed. If clinical signs of anthrax occur, empiric therapy for anthrax is indicated, pending definitive diagnosis. Optimally, patients should have medical care available upon discontinuation of antibiotics from a fixed medical care facility with intensive care capabilities and infectious disease consultants.

---

*Partially vaccinated = patients who have received <5 intramuscular priming doses or have not received all annual boosters

** Fully vaccinated = patients who have completed the five dose intramuscular series and are up to date on all annual boosters

Brucellosis

SUMMARY

Signs and Symptoms: When present, include fever, headache, myalgias, arthralgias, back pain, profuse sweats, chills, weight loss, and generalized malaise. Onset may be acute or insidious. Fever may be intermittent or continuous and recurrences are common even after antibiotic treatment. Subclinical infections have been reported. The osteoarticular complications of brucellosis occur commonly, particularly sacroiliitis, and can produce significant disability. Other manifestations include depression and other mental status changes, epididymoorchitis, and localized suppurative organ infection. Morbidity may be pronounced, but fatalities are uncommon.

Diagnosis: Diagnosis requires a high index of suspicion, as most infections present as non-specific febrile illnesses or are asymptomatic. Laboratory diagnosis can be made by serum agglutination tests, ELISA, immunofluorescence, and by standard culture. Blood cultures often require extended incubation to become positive, even up to 30 days. Bone marrow cultures may produce a higher yield. Other body fluids may be tested depending on infection distribution (synovial, pleural, CSF).

Treatment: Antibiotic therapy with doxycycline and rifampin (or other medications) for 6 weeks is sufficient in most cases. More prolonged regimens may be required for patients with complications such as hepatitis, splenitis, meningoencephalitis, endocarditis, or osteomyelitis.

Prophylaxis: A human vaccine is not available. Prophylaxis should only be considered for high-risk exposure in the following situations: (1) inadvertent wound or mucous membrane exposure to infected livestock tissues and body fluids and to livestock vaccines, (2) exposure to laboratory aerosols or to secondary aerosols generated from contaminated soil particles in calving and lambing areas, (3) confirmed biowarfare exposure.

Isolation and Decontamination: Brucellosis is spread readily via bodily fluids and aerosols. Standard precautions are appropriate for healthcare workers. If an attack with *Brucella* sp. is suspected, special care should be taken to avoid the generation of secondary aerosols. Person-to-person transmission has occasionally been reported by tissue transplantation and sexual contact. Contact surfaces that are free of organic matter can be decontaminated with a 0.5% hypochlorite solution; higher concentrations (>5%), or other disinfectants for gram-negative microorganisms, should be used where organic matter cannot be effectively reduced or controlled.

OVERVIEW

Brucellosis is an important disease of livestock in many countries and is caused by infection with one of several species of *Brucella*, a group of gram-negative cocco-baccilli that are facultative intracellular pathogens (Table 1). It likely has a worldwide distribution, but accurate surveillance data are not available in some countries.

Brucellosis is primarily a disease of the reproductive system of livestock and, depending on the species affected, is associated with infertility, abortion, retained fetal membranes, orchitis, and infection of the male accessory sex glands. Transmission in most livestock is primarily by ingestion of organisms either shed from or contaminated with fetal membranes, aborted fetuses, and uterine discharges, and occasionally from dams to nursing young. *Brucellae* also enter the body through mucous membranes, conjunctivae, wounds, and occasionally through intact skin.

TABLE 1. Characteristics of brucellosis infection in livestock and humans

Brucella spp.	1° Reservoir	2° Hosts	Geographic Distribution	Human Exposure Activity	Pathogenicity To Humans
Abortus	Cattle, Bison, Deer	Goat, Sheep, Dog, Human	Worldwide	Raw dairy foods, animal husbandry, laboratory	Moderate
Melitensis	Goat, Sheep	Dog, Human	Latin America, Asia, Mediterranean	Raw dairy foods, animal husbandry, laboratory	Highest
Suis	Pig (feral, and domestic)	Dog, Human, Cattle	SE Asia, Scattered and Midwest US, S America	Pork slaughter, processing, feral pig hunting, laboratory	High
Canis	Dog, Coyote		Scattered	Dog breeding and whelping	Moderate

Zoonotic transmission to humans has occurred by contact with infected tissues and discharges (aborted fetuses, fetal membranes and vaginal discharges), blood, urine, and semen. Veterinarians, slaughterhouse workers, ranchers, and other livestock husbandry workers and hunters have been infected in occupational and recreational settings. Transmission to humans also occurs by ingesting raw milk and other dairy products from infected animals. Though less common, airborne infections have also occurred in livestock husbandry settings (inhalation of contaminated particles from soil and bedding in birthing areas) and in laboratory settings. Finally, accidental percutaneous exposure to modified-live livestock vaccines (e.g., veterinarians) has also occurred. The *Brucella* species associated with human infection are: *B. abortus*, *B. melitensis*, *B. suis*, and, rarely, *B. canis* (Table 1).

It is estimated that inhalation of only 10 to 100 bacteria is sufficient to cause disease in humans. Subclinical infections are relatively common. Brucellosis has a low case fatality rate (5% of untreated cases), with rare deaths caused by complications such as endocarditis or meningitis. When disease is naturally occurring, the incubation period may be several days to several months. However, large aerosol doses (as would be expected in a biowarfare scenario) would shorten the incubation period, lead to higher clinical attack rates, and result in more prolonged, incapacitating, and disabling disease than in its natural form.

HISTORY AND SIGNIFICANCE

Marston described disease manifestations caused by *B. melitensis* (Mediterranean fever, gastric intermittent fever) among British soldiers on Malta during the Crimean War. Goats were identified as the source. Restrictions on the consumption of unpasteurized dairy goat products soon decreased the incidence among military personnel. *B. abortus* was first isolated by Bruce and described by Bang and Stribolt in 1897. Synonyms for human brucellosis vary by region and include undulant fever, Malta fever, rock fever, Gibraltar fever, melitoccie goat fever, Texas fever, Rio Grande fever, Bang fever and Brucella fever. In 1954, *B. suis* became the first agent weaponized by the U.S. at its Pine Bluff Arsenal located in Arkansas. *Brucella* species survive well in aerosols and resist drying.

Human brucellosis is now a rare disease in the U.S. with about 100 cases per yr reported. Most are reported from CA, FL, TX, and VA, and the majority of these are associated with ingestion of unpasteurized dairy products made outside of the U.S. and privately imported (thus escaping FDA and

USDA regulatory food-safety initiatives). Rare infections may still occur in meat processing or livestock handling settings in areas with herds or flocks that are not certified 'brucellosis-free' by regional animal health authorities. Human brucellosis is highly endemic in some Mediterranean basin and Arabian peninsular countries, as well as India, Mexico, South and Central America and many of the republics of the former Soviet Union. Disease incidence and prevalence vary regionally, with some reporting annual incidences of over 80 cases per 100,000 population. Serologic evidence of *Brucella* spp. exposure on an Arabian peninsular country was near 20% with more than 2% having active disease (WHO). A few regions in Kuwait have reported annual incidences as high as 128 cases per 100,000 population. These highlight a risk to military personnel in the region.

CLINICAL FEATURES

Brucellosis is a systemic disease that can involve any organ system and can present in a variety of clinical manifestations. Untreated, *Brucella* localizes in the reticuloendothelial system organs, primarily the liver, spleen, and bone marrow, where granuloma formation ensues. Large granulomas serve as a source for persistent bacteremia.

The incubation period is typically 3-4 wks, but can range from 1 wk to many months. Illness can present suddenly, over a few days, or insidiously over weeks to months. Patients usually complain of non-specific symptoms such as fever (90-95%), malaise (80-95%), sweats (40-90%), and myalgias/arthralgias (40-70%). Other common symptoms include fatigue, chills, and backache. Fever is usually intermittent, and can assume an undulant (wavelike) pattern in patients with chronic, untreated infection. Neuropsychiatric symptoms including depression, headache, and irritability, are common. Gastrointestinal symptoms (abdominal pain, anorexia, constipation, diarrhea, vomiting) are reported in nearly 70% of adult cases. Cough, dyspnea, chest pain, and testicular pain can occur less frequently. Common physical signs include hepatomegaly (10-70%) and/or splenomegaly (10-30%), arthritis (up to 40%), weight loss, and adenopathy (10-20%).

Osteoarticular complications including bursitis, tenosynovitis, arthritis, osteomyelitis, sacroiliitis, discitis, and paravertebral abscess are reported in 20-60% of brucellosis cases. Sacroiliitis typically presents acutely with fever and focal lower back pain and occurs in up to 30% of cases, predominantly in young men. Arthritis of large, weight-bearing joints of the lower extremities may occur in 20% of cases. Arthritis is usually monoarticular, but can be polyarticular up to 30% of the time. Spondylitis or vertebral osteomyelitis may affect from up to 30% of all cases of brucellosis. Patients with spondylitis tend to be older and have a more chronic, destructive disease course than those with sacroiliitis or peripheral arthritis; the lumbar vertebrae are most commonly affected.

Gastrointestinal disease can manifest as ileitis, colitis, or granulomatous or mononuclear infiltrative hepatitis. Hepatitis only progresses to cirrhosis if pre-existing liver disease (e.g., hepatitis C or alcoholic liver disease) is present. Pulmonary disease may be present in 1 to 5% of cases and may take the form of lung abscess, single or miliary nodules, bronchopneumonia, enlarged hilar lymph nodes, or pleural effusions. While inhalational exposure to *Brucella* has been described in laboratory or abattoir workers, this route of infection has not proven to lead with regularity to any particular form of disease (e.g., pneumonic).

Epididymoorchitis has been described in 2-20% of male patients with brucellosis. They typically present acutely with scrotal pain and swelling, and continuous fever. Orchitis is unilateral in the majority of cases.

Neurologic disease can take the form of meningitis, encephalitis, peripheral neuropathy, brain or epidural abscesses, radiculoneuropathies or meningovascular syndromes. However, direct CNS invasion occurs in less than 5% of cases of brucellosis. Behavioral disturbances and psychoses appear to occur unrelated to the degree of fever and may be only occasionally associated with the aforementioned syndromes during acute phases.

Endocarditis occurs in less than 2% of cases, but accounts for the majority of brucellosis-related deaths.

Acute brucellosis during the first 2 trimesters of pregnancy has been reported to lead to spontaneous abortion in up to 40% of cases if untreated, while untreated disease may be associated with intrauterine fetal death in only 2% of cases with onset in the third trimester.

Disease type and severity may vary with the infecting *Brucella* species. *B. melitensis* is the most pathogenic; human infection is associated with an acute course and disabling complications. *B. suis* infection is associated with localized abscess formation and a chronic course. *B. abortus* and *B. canis* infections are associated with frequent relapses and insidious onset.

DIAGNOSIS

A high index of suspicion is necessary to initiate the appropriate testing and ultimately diagnose and treat brucellosis. Animal contact history, consumption of unpasteurized dairy products (including goat), and travel to endemic areas should prompt consideration of brucellosis. It should be suspected when a patient presents with acute or insidious onset of fever, night sweats, undue fatigue, GI symptoms, anorexia, weight loss, headache, arthralgias and splenomegaly, and / or hepatomegaly. Additionally, patients with some of the aforementioned complications, such as sacroiliitis or epididymoorchitis should be tested for brucellosis when appropriate. Brucellosis is occasionally diagnosed in patients with non-specific symptoms who have been previously evaluated for many other etiologies, and a thorough review of risk factors detects a potential exposure to *Brucella* species.

The leukocyte count in brucellosis patients is usually normal but may be low; anemia, neutropenia, and thrombocytopenia may occur in a minority of cases. AST and ALT may be mildly elevated, and erythrocyte sedimentation rate (ESR) is normal or only mildly elevated in the majority of cases.

Imaging studies may help to identify localized infection. Persistent fever after therapy or the prolonged presence of significant musculoskeletal complaints should prompt CT or MR imaging. ^{99m}Technetium and ^{67}gallium scans are reasonably sensitive means for detecting sacroiliitis and other axial skeletal infections. CXR may be unremarkable even with respiratory symptoms. Cranial CT scan may be useful for patients with neurologic signs or deficits. Though this study is also often normal, occasional leptomeningitis, cerebral abscess, or other pathology may be identified. Echocardiography may reveal evidence of endocarditis. Vegetative lesions are most common on the aortic valve (sinus of Valsalva), followed by the mitral valve. Testicular ultrasound may be helpful in distinguishing *Brucella* epididymoorchitis from testicular abscess or tumor.

There are three categories of tests that are usually employed for the diagnosis of brucellosis when available: culture, serologic testing, immunoflourescence (IF) and molecular diagnostics. Each modality has limitations. Blood cultures are typically negative in patients taking antibiotics. In many countries, antibiotics can easily be obtained without a prescription, and are frequently obtained by patients before presentation to healthcare facilities. The utilization of serologic testing is the most common diagnostic test utilized for brucellosis worldwide in the form of agglutination tests. These tests can often give false-positive results in endemic areas, as patients may have been remotely exposed to brucellosis. Agglutination test results can also be problematic in patients with relapsed infection. IF can only be utilized when a biopsy of infected tissue is obtained. Molecular diagnostics, usually with PCR platforms, can have false-negative results, possibly due to inhibitors of PCR in the patient's blood. Because all modalities have limitations, multiple categories of tests may be conducted to establish the diagnosis.

Brucella species are small, non-motile, non-encapsulated, non-spore forming, slow-growing, coccobacilli gram-negative intracellular aerobes. While formerly cultures were held for many weeks to show growth, automated blood culture systems will grow *Brucellae* within 7 d in 95% of cases. However, rapid identification systems may misidentify the organism, often as *Psychrobacter phenylpyruvicus*. If traditional, non-automated blood culture is performed, a biphasic culture method (e.g., Castaneda bottle) may improve the chances of isolation, as may re-culture onto solid medium every week for 2 mos. Clinically, identification to the genus level is adequate to initiate therapy. Speciation is epidemiologically necessary and helps to inform prognosis; however, it requires more specialized analyses.

Blood and bone marrow cultures taken during the acute febrile phase of illness yield the organism in 15-70 % and 92% of cases, respectively. Other fluid cultures are encouraged in accordance with accompanying clinical signs (CSF with meningitis, joint fluid with effusion, urine with genitourinary signs). Bone marrow and liver biopsies (to detect granulomatous disease) may also be indicated. Clinical laboratories should always be alerted if a diagnosis of brucellosis is suspected. This permits the use of selective isolation media and the implementation of BSL-3 containment.

Diagnostic laboratory criteria include: 1) isolation of *Brucella* sp. from a clinical specimen; 2) at least a fourfold rise in *Brucella* sp. agglutination titer between acute and convalescent sera obtained at least 2 wks apart and performed at the same laboratory; 3) demonstration by IF of *Brucella* sp. in a clinical specimen. A <u>probable case</u> is one that is clinically compatible and epidemiologically linked to a confirmed case or that has supportive serology (i.e., *Brucella* agglutination titer of at least 1:160 in one or more serum specimens obtained after onset of symptoms). A <u>confirmed case</u> is a clinically compatible case that is laboratory confirmed.

A serum agglutination test (SAT) for IgM and IgG, and a tube agglutination method for anti-O polysaccharide antibody is available; titers of at least 1:160 by each indicate active disease. ELISA is also available. CSF and joint fluid may also be used for antibody testing with some test kits.

MEDICAL MANAGEMENT

Historically, the most effective proven treatment for acute brucellosis in adults is the combination of oral doxycycline 100 mg bid for 4-6 wks plus streptomycin 1 g IM daily for the first 2-3 wks. If streptomycin is not available, gentamicin probably represents a suitable alternative. For uncomplicated acute brucellosis, combinations of oral antibiotics are usually sufficient, or even preferred, as they are simpler to use in the outpatient setting and have comparable cure rates to doxycycline-aminoglycoside combinations. The most widely recommended combination for adults and children over 8 yrs old is doxycycline (100 mg PO bid for adults, 2.2 mg/kg PO bid (up to 200 mg/d) for children) + rifampin (600-900 mg/d PO qd for adults,15-20 mg/kg (up to 600-900 mg/d) for children) for 4-6 weeks; a fluoroquinolone (e.g., ofloxacin or ciprofloxacin) + rifampin or trimethoprim-sulfamethoxazole (TMP-SMX) + rifampin may be appropriate alternatives. Relapse rates are 5-10% for most combination oral regimens and higher for monotherapy (up to 30% with TMP-SMX alone). During pregnancy and for children < 8 yrs old, the combination of TMP-SMX and rifampin has usually been preferred, as doxycycline poses a potential risk to the fetus or young child's skeletal and dental development.

Acute, complicated brucellosis (e.g., skeletal disease, endocarditis) often requires long-term triple-drug therapy for effective cure. A combination of oral rifampin and doxycycline (or TMP-SMX in children < 8 yrs old), plus IM streptomycin (or gentamicin) for the first 2-3 weeks has been used most frequently. For skeletal disease, 6-8 wks of antibiotics may be necessary for cure; persisting musculoskeletal complaints may be present in patients with chronic infection and sacroiliitis. Meningoencephalitis and endocarditis should receive at least 90 days of therapy and may require > 6 months. Endocarditis typically responds poorly to antibiotics alone and generally requires surgical excision of the affected valve. Necrotizing orchitis and other suppurative complications of brucellosis may require surgical excision or drainage.

Patient education is a critical component of medical management and must include emphasis on the importance of antibiotic compliance.

Periodic follow-up is also critical, and referral to medical specialists may be indicated. As is the case with all bacterial bioagents, antibiotic resistance can be engineered into the organism, and thus determination of antibiotic susceptibilities in an intentional attack with *Brucella* is paramount.

Infection control. Standard precautions are adequate in managing brucellosis patients, as the disease is not generally transmissible from person-to-person. Mask, gloves, and eye protection are indicated for respiratory procedures and for handling body fluids. BSL-3 containment practices should be used when handling suspected *Brucella* sp. cultures in the laboratory because of potential aerosol exposure.

PROPHYLAXIS

The risk of foodborne brucellosis is reduced by avoiding unpasteurized dairy products particularly while traveling in areas where brucellosis occurs in livestock. Travelers should consult with animal health and public health authorities before travel to assess the foodborne and endemic brucellosis risks. Most developed countries have largely eradicated brucellosis from domestic cattle herds and sheep and goat flocks by multifaceted control programs. These may include periodic testing and slaughter of positive and contact animals and periodic batch testing of raw milk. Livestock vaccines are available and are tightly controlled by regional animal health authorities. No licensed human brucellosis vaccine is available.

Despite extensive studies, optimal antibiotic therapy for brucellosis remains under dispute. The CDC interim PEP recommendations for high-risk exposures to *Brucella* are: doxycycline 100 mg PO bid plus rifampin 600 mg qd PO. Brucellosis is a reportable human and livestock disease in the U.S. and many other countries.

Glanders and Melioidosis

SUMMARY

Symptoms and signs: Incubation periods after inhalation are usually less than 14 d, but may range from days to weeks for glanders and days to decades for melioidosis. Onset of symptoms may be abrupt or gradual. Respiratory tract disease can produce fever (usually above 102°F), rigors, sweats, myalgias, headache, pleuritic chest pain, and cervical lymphadenopathy. Pneumonia can progress rapidly and result in bacteremia, sepsis, and disseminated infection, leading to hepatosplenomegaly and generalized papular/pustular eruptions. Both diseases are usually fatal without treatment.

Diagnosis: Methylene blue or Wright's stain of exudates may reveal scant small bacilli with a safety-pin bipolar appearance. Standard cultures can identify both *Burkholderia mallei* and *B. pseudomallei* (the causative agents of glanders and melioidosis, respectively). CXR may show infiltrates with consolidation and cavitation, multiple small lung abscess, or miliary lesions. Abdominal ultrasound may reveal splenic or hepatic abscesses. Leukocyte counts may be normal, elevated, or decreased. Serologic tests may be useful, but low titers or negative serology does not exclude the diagnosis.

Treatment: Initial therapy consists of the IV administration of either ceftazidime, imipenem, or meropenem (plus trimethoprim-sulfamethoxazole (TMP-SMX) if septicemic), followed by prolonged oral antibiotic therapy. Surgical drainage is indicated for large abscesses. Life-long follow-up is advised after treatment for melioidosis due to a risk of relapse.

Prophylaxis: No vaccines are currently available. There are no human data or FDA-approved regimens for postexposure prophylaxis, although TMP-SMX shows promise in animal studies, and should be given ASAP after exposure. Additional information can be found in the *Glanders & Melioidosis* section of Appendix D. Bioagent Vaccines, Prohylaxis, and Therapeutics.

Isolation and Decontamination: Person-to-person airborne or droplet transmission is unlikely, although secondary cases may occur through improper handling of infectious materials. Standard precautions for healthcare workers. Contact precautions are indicated while caring for patients with skin lesions. Cultures must be managed under BSL-3 conditions. Environmental decontamination using a 0.5%-1.0% hypochlorite solution should be effective.

OVERVIEW

The etiologic agents of glanders and melioidosis are *Burkholderia mallei* and *Burkholderia pseudomallei*, respectively. Both are gram-negative bacilli which may have a "safety-pin" appearance on methylene blue or Wright's stain.

B. mallei persists in nature only in infected animal hosts, and causes disease in horses, mules, and donkeys. Human cases have occurred among veterinarians, horse and donkey caretakers, and abattoir workers. In the past, humans seldom became infected, despite frequent and often close contact with infected animals. This may be due to exposure to low concentrations of organisms from infected sites in ill animals and because strains virulent for equids are often less virulent for humans. The low transmission rates of *B. mallei* to humans from infected horses is exemplified by the fact that in China, during World War II, 30% of tested horses were positive for glanders, but human cases were rare. Both acute and chronic disease may develop in animals and humans. Acute presentations are more common in mules and donkeys, with death typically occurring within 3-4 wks. Chronic disease is more common in horses and humans, and causes multiple skin nodules that ulcerate and drain, and induration, enlargement, and nodular lesions of superficial lymphatic vessels of the extremities, regional lymphadenopathy, and abscesses of internal organs. The cutaneous and lymphatic disease in horses is known as "farcy."

B. pseudomallei is widely distributed in water and soil in many tropical and subtropical regions. The organism can be isolated from 50% of rice paddies in Thailand. *B. pseudomallei* spreads to humans by inoculation of nasal, oral, or conjunctival mucous membranes, abraded or lacerated skin, or by inhalation. Melioidosis is endemic in southeast Asia and northern Australia, where it is most prevalent during the rainy season among people who have direct contact with wet soils. Most exposed individuals do not develop symptomatic melioidosis; many people in endemic regions asymptomatically seroconvert to *B. pseudomallei* early in life. Most (50-70%) of those who develop symptomatic disease have predisposing medical conditions including diabetes mellitus (present in up to 50% of cases), alcoholism, cirrhosis, renal disease, thallassemia, cystic fibrosis, or impaired immunity. Clinical presentations vary from mild disease to overwhelming septicemia with up to a 90% case fatality rate (CFR) and death within

24-48 h after onset. Melioidosis can also reactivate years after primary infection and result in chronic and life-threatening disease.

Aerosols from cultures are highly infectious to laboratory workers. BSL-3 containment practices are required when working with cultures of these organisms. Clinical chemistries, hematology, and other laboratory tests may be done under BSL- 2 conditions. Person-to-person spread is rare. Because of their potential transmission by environmental aerosols, virulence, difficult treatment regimens and the lack of available vaccines, *B. mallei* and *B. pseudomallei* have been viewed as potential bioagents.

HISTORY AND SIGNIFICANCE

B. mallei was reportedly one of the first bacterial agents to be weaponized in a modern biological warfare program. During World War I, a German agent in Baltimore allegedly inoculated horses, mules and donkeys intended for export to Allied forces in Europe. The intent was to disrupt troop and supply convoys. The effectiveness of these alleged biological attacks is unknown. The Japanese deliberately infected horses, civilians, and prisoners of war with *B. mallei* at the Pinfang Institute in occupied China during World War II. The U.S. studied this agent as a possible biowarfare weapon in 1943-44 but did not weaponize it. The Soviet Union is believed to have identified *B. mallei* as a potential bioagent after World War II. Despite the efficiency of laboratory transmission, glanders has only been sporadic in humans, and no epidemics of human disease have been reported. There have been no naturally acquired cases of human glanders in the U.S. since 1942. Sporadic cases still occur in Asia, Africa, the Middle East, and South America.

Melioidosis is a leading cause of community-acquired bacterial pneumonia and sepsis in northern Australia, and has accounted for 20% of community-acquired bacterial sepsis in northern Thailand. Pulmonary melioidosis occurred among US forces during the Viet Nam conflict, thought to have been due to inhalation of aerosols of contaminated soil and water generated by helicopter prop blast in irrigated rice fields. As a result of *B. pseudomallei's* potentially long incubation period, French and later U.S. soldiers returning from Viet Nam would infrequently develop disease (the "Vietnamese time-bomb") years after exposure. *B. pseudomallei* was also studied by the U.S. as a potential bioagent, but never weaponized. It has been reported that the Soviet Union also evaluated *B. pseudomallei* as a bioagent.

CLINICAL FEATURES

The manifestations of both glanders and melioidosis are protean; disease can be localized or systemic, acute or chronic, or progress from one form to another over time. Inhalation of aerosols produced by a biowarfare weapon containing high inocula of *B. mallei* or *B. pseudomallei* could presumably produce any of these syndromes, although acute respiratory or systemic syndromes would be the most likely.

Incubation periods vary by route of entry, size of inoculum, virulence of the organism, and host factors. Animal models of high dose inhalational exposure to either *B. mallei or B. pseudomallei* result in incubation periods that are usually 1-4 d. In the few well-documented cases of human glanders due to respiratory exposure, the incubation period varied from 10-14 d. Mucus membrane or skin exposure led to symptoms within 1-5 d (range 1-21 d). The incubation period of naturally acquired melioidosis is more difficult to determine, because environmental exposure to the agent in endemic regions may be continuous. Documented incubation periods for clinically overt melioidosis are typically 1-21 d, although prolonged incubation periods of months to decades can occur. Uncommonly, patients may present with active meliodosis more than 20 yrs after exposure, usually after the onset of diabetes or other risk factors.

Acute glanders and melioidosis after intentional high-titer aerosol exposure can be expected to be clinically indistinguishable; differentiation will depend heavily upon laboratory studies. Pneumonia would likely develop. Patients would likely present within a few days of exposure with acute onset of fever, chills, malaise, fatigue, myalgias, and shortness of breath, with or without cough and pleuritic chest pain. Cough is likely to become productive, and hemoptysis is possible. CXR findings vary and may disclose unilateral or bilateral, multifocal, nodular, or lobar consolidation, often progressing to abscess formation and cavitation. Failure to provide prompt therapy is likely to lead to fulminant sepsis, shock, and multi-organ system failure. Metastatic septic foci may develop, with hepatic, splenic, and cutaneous abscesses being the most likely, although any organ can be affected.

The clinical course of these illnesses may suggest other biological-agent related diseases in the differential diagnosis. A rapidly progressive pneumonia accompanied by clinical sepsis, with respiratory secretions demonstrating gram-negative bacteria with "safety pin" appearance on Wright's stain suggests pneumonic plague, while a diffuse papular or pustular rash may suggest smallpox.

Natural disease due to both organisms is well-described in the literature. Differences between the clinical presentations of glanders and melioidosis may result from mucocutaneous or low inoculum exposures, and are described below.

Glanders. Cutaneous exposure typically leads to local inflammatory nodules with subsequent lymphangitis (sometimes with sporotrichoid nodule distribution) and regional lymphadenitis. Nodules typically ulcerate and drain. Conjunctival involvement can result in photophobia, lacrimation, and purulent discharge. Constitutional symptoms may be acute or subacute, and include fever (may be low-grade or recurring), rigors, sweats, headache, fatigue and myalgias.

Inhalational exposure may produce either upper or lower respiratory tract disease. Pharyngitis or rhinitis may feature constitutional symptoms, headache, purulent exudates, and cervical lymphadenopathy. Chronic infection and erosion of the nasal septum and turbinates can lead to severe disfigurement. Pulmonary involvement may follow inhalation of organisms or develop secondarily by hematogenous spread, and may be rapidly progressive.

Septicemia may occur at any time during the disease, regardless of the mode of entry. Sepsis can feature tachycardia, jaundice, and diarrhea. Bacteremia may result in diffuse seeding of the skin, leading to a regional or generalized papular and/or pustular rash that may be mistaken for smallpox. Disseminated infection may produce granulomatous lesions and abscesses of internal organs (especially liver, spleen, and lungs) and skeletal muscles. These abscesses may result in hepatosplenomegaly and abdominal tenderness. Osteomyelitis, brain abscess, and meningitis have been reported. Disseminated infection carries a high risk of rapidly progressive septic shock and death.

Chronic disease occurs in half of all natural cases and is eventually fatal without treatment. Chronic infections may feature spontaneous clinical remission followed by relapse. CFRs dropped to 20% for localized disease, and to 40% overall, after sulfadiazine therapy became available. Treatment experience using modern antibiotics is, however, limited.

Melioidosis. Mucocutaneous exposure may lead to local nodules / abscesses and regional lymphadenitis. Cutaneous disease may result from local inoculation, or from spread to the skin through the bloodstream. Rarely, melioidosis will present as a distal, focal abscess with or without an obvious site of primary inoculation; most commonly as a primary purulent parotitis in children (more common in Thailand) or as a primary prostatic abscess (more common in northern Australia).

Inhalational exposure, either through near drowning or via infectious aerosols, may result in an acute respiratory disease which can range from a mild bronchitis to a chronic subacute pneumonia, or a severe acute necrotizing pneumonia and septic shock. Sputum is often purulent, and hemoptysis may be present. Radiographic findings commonly feature lobar or segmental consolidation with a predilection for the upper lobes, or multiple, widespread 0.5-1.0 cm nodules, or cavitation. Chronic pulmonary disease can follow acute pulmonary disease, or reactivate years after exposure, with clinical and radiographic findings similar to those of tuberculosis.

Up to 60% of patients, particularly those with risk factors, become bacteremic. Septicemic melioidosis presents with fever, rigors, night sweats, myalgia, anorexia, and headache. Additional features can include papular or pustular skin lesions, diarrhea, and hepatosplenomegaly. Dissemination is likely to produce cutaneous and internal (especially liver and spleen) abscesses even weeks to months later. Prostatic abscess occurs in 2-15% of cases. Poor prognostic indicators for severe melioidosis include positive blood cultures within 24 h of incubation and neutropenia. Without proper treatment, most septicemic patients will die within 2-3 d. With treatment, overall mortality for severe melioidosis is up to 50% in Thailand and 19% in Australia. Relapse is common, even after prolonged antimicrobial therapy.

DIAGNOSIS

Microbiology. Gram stain of lesion exudates reveals small irregularly staining, gram-negative bacilli. Methylene blue or Wright's stain may reveal bipolar "safety pin" staining. The organisms can be cultured from abscesses/wounds, secretions, sputum (in pneumonia), and sometimes blood and urine with standard bacteriological media; adding 1-5% glucose, 5% glycerol, or meat infusion nutrient agar may accelerate growth. Primary isolation requires 48-72 h in agar at 37.5° C; automated blood culture methods are typically more rapid. *B. pseudomallei* is generally more rapidly growing and less fastidious than *B. mallei*. Selective media (e.g., Ashdown's medium for *B. pseudomallei*) may be necessary for isolation from non-sterile sites (sputum, pharyngeal cultures).

Blood cultures for *B. mallei* are <u>rarely</u> positive. In contrast, blood cultures for *B. pseudomallei* are <u>often</u> positive and urine culture may be positive, especially if prostatitis or renal abscesses are present. Cultures must be performed under BSL-3 precautions due to the high aerosol risk these agents pose to laboratory workers.

Specific, rapid immunoassays may be available in some reference laboratories for *B. pseudomallei* capsular antigens. PCR is sensitive and specific, but available in only a few reference laboratories.

Serology. For *B. mallei*, agglutination tests are not positive for at least 7-10 d (sometimes up to 3 wks), and a high background titer in normal sera (1:320 to 1:640) makes interpretation difficult. Complement fixation (CF) tests are more specific, but less sensitive, and may require 40 d for conversion. CF tests are considered positive if the titer is equal to, or exceeds 1:20. For *B. pseudomallei*, a fourfold increase in titer supports the diagnosis of melioidosis. A single IgM titer above 1:160 with a compatible clinical picture suggests active infection; IgG is less useful in endemic regions due to high seroprevalence.

Other laboratory studies. In septicemic glanders, mild leukocytosis with a shift to the left or leukopenia with a relative lymphocytosis may occur. In systemic melioidosis, significant leukocytosis with left shift is common, and leucopenia / neutropenia are poor prognostic indicators; anemia, coagulopathy, and evidence of hepatic or renal dysfunction may be present.

Radiographic studies. CXRs may demonstrate lobar or segmental opacification, or diffuse nodular opacities. Cavitary lesions are common, but effusions and hilar adenopathy are rare. Abdominal and pelvic computerized tomography (CT) scans or ultrasounds should be considered for all patients with suspected glanders or melioidosis to exclude hepatic, splenic or prostatic abscesses. Prostatic abscess in melioidosis can be delineated as a heterogeneous multiloculated fluid collection within an enlarged prostate, using transrectal ultrasound, CT, or magnetic resonance (MR) imaging.

Pathology. Pathologic tissue findings may feature granulomatous lesions resembling tuberculosis. This similarity can make diagnosis difficult, especially in areas where both melioidosis and tuberculosis are endemic, such as Thailand.

MEDICAL MANAGEMENT

Supportive Care. Ventilatory support may be necessary for severe pulmonary disease. Septicemic patients often require aggressive supportive care including fluid resuscitation, vasopressors, and management of coagulopathy. Large abscesses and empyemas should be drained when possible; prostatic and parotid abscesses in patients with melioidosis are unlikely to resolve without surgical intervention. Surgical therapy is not necessary for multiple small hepatic or splenic abscesses, which respond to prolonged antibiotic therapy.

Antimicrobials. Antibiotic regimens for melioidosis are based on clinical trials and medical experience in Thailand and Australia. Although clinical experience with human glanders is limited due to its low incidence during the antibiotic era, the same treatment regimens are recommended for both diseases. *B. mallei* and *B. pseudomallei* have similar antibiotic susceptibility patterns (although, unlike *B. pseudomallei*, natural *B. mallei* strains generally remain susceptible to aminoglycosides and macrolides in vitro). Revision of empiric regimens is guided by antibiotic susceptibilities of bacterial isolates as determined by the clinical laboratory.

Initial therapy. All cases of both diseases, regardless of clinical severity, should be treated initially with IV therapy for at least 2 wks, followed by oral eradication therapy for at least another 3 mos. Antibiotic regimens include either ceftazidime (120 mg/kg/d IV in three divided doses), imipenem (60 mg/kg/d IV in four divided doses, max 4 gm/d), or meropenem (75 mg/kg/d IV in three divided doses, max 6 gm/d). Many experts add TMP/SMX (TMP 8 mg/kg/d IV in four divided doses); oral TMP/SMX has been substituted when the IV formulation was not available. If ceftazidime or a carbapenem are not available, ampicillin/sulbactam or other intravenous beta-lactam/beta-lactamase inhibitor combinations may represent viable, albeit less-proven alternatives. IV antibiotics should be continued for at least 14 d and until the patient shows clinical improvement. IV therapy may be extended for critical illness, severe pulmonary disease, deep-seated abscesses, bone, joint, or CNS involvement. Patients may remain febrile for prolonged periods during appropriate antimicrobial therapy. Median time to fever resolution is 9 d, but can be significantly longer in patients with large, undrained abscesses.

Septic shock. Australian researchers have combined IV antibiotics with granulocyte colony-stimulating factor (G-CSF) 300 g IV per d for 10 d (or longer if clinical shock persists) in melioidosis patients with septic shock. Mortality dropped from a historic rate of 95% to 10% with G-CSF; however, limitations in the study preclude attributing success entirely to G-CSF. Further studies are warranted to determine its role in treatment.

Maintenance therapy. Upon completion of IV therapy, oral maintenance therapy should be continued for at least 3-6 mos. Maintenance therapy of severe disease should continue for at least 20 wks to reduce the rate of relapse to less than 10%; however, longer courses (6-12 months) may be necessary depending upon response to therapy and severity of initial illness (e.g., longer courses for extrapulmonary suppurative disease). Historically, maintenance therapy combined four oral drugs (doxycycline and TMP/SMX for at least 20 weeks, plus chloramphenicol for the first 8 weeks); but side effects were common and compliance was poor. Equivalent results have been obtained with doxycycline (100 mg PO bid) plus TMP/SMX (4 mg/kg/d in two divided doses) for 20 wks. Amoxicillin/clavulanic acid has been used in some cases and may be the antibiotic of choice during pregnancy or for children less than 8 yrs old. Combinations including fluoroquinolones show promise, but have not been validated. Lifelong follow-up is indicated for melioidosis patients to identify relapse.

Isolation precautions. Person-to-person airborne or respiratory droplet transmission is unlikely, although secondary cases may occur through improper handling of infectious materials. Standard precautions should be used to prevent person-to-person transmission in proven or suspected cases. Contact precautions are indicated while caring for patients with skin involvement. Droplet or airborne precautions should be used, respectively, if pneumonic plague or pulmonary tuberculosis are considerations in the differential diagnosis. Environmental decontamination using a 0.5%-1.0% hypochlorite solution is effective.

PROPHYLAXIS

Vaccine: There are currently no vaccines available for human use.

Antibiotics: There are no human data or FDA-approved postexposure prophylaxis regimens for these diseases. TMP-SMX has been effective in limited animal studies. Ciprofloxacin and doxycycline have been associated with high relapse rates in animals. Optimum duration of prophylaxis is unknown, but at least 10 d should be considered.

Plague

SUMMARY

Signs and Symptoms: Pneumonic plague begins with sudden onset of symptoms after an incubation period of 1-6 d. Symptoms include high fever, chills, headache, malaise, followed by cough (often with hemoptysis), progressing rapidly to dyspnea, stridor, cyanosis, and death. Gastrointestinal symptoms are often present. Death results from respiratory failure, circulatory collapse, and a bleeding diathesis. Bubonic plague is characterized by swollen painful lymph nodes called buboes (often in the inguinal area), high fever, and malaise. Bubonic plague may progress spontaneously to the septicemic form (septic shock, thrombosis, disseminated intravascular coagulation) or to the pneumonic form. Plague meningitis is also possible.

Diagnosis: Suspect plague if large numbers of previously healthy individuals suddenly develop severe pneumonia, especially if hemoptysis is present with gram-negative coccobacilli in sputum. Presumptive diagnosis can be made by Gram, Wright, Giemsa, or Wayson stain of blood, sputum, CSF, or lymph node aspirates. Definitive diagnosis requires culture of the organism from those sites. Immunodiagnosis is helpful in establishing a presumptive diagnosis.

Treatment: Early administration of antibiotics is critical, as pneumonic plague is invariably fatal if it is delayed more than 1 d after the onset of symptoms. The treatment of choice is parenteral streptomycin or gentamicin, with doxycycline or ciprofloxacin representing alternatives. Duration of therapy is at least 10-14 d. For plague meningitis, add chloramphenicol to the regimen.

Prophylaxis: For asymptomatic persons exposed to a plague aerosol or to a suspected pneumonic plague case, doxycycline 100 mg is given PO bid for 7 d or for the duration of risk of exposure plus 1 wk. Alternative antibiotics include ciprofloxacin, tetracycline, or chloramphenicol. No vaccine is currently available for plague prophylaxis. The previously available licensed, killed vaccine (manufactured by Greer) was effective against natural bubonic plague, but not against aerosol exposure. No prophylaxis is required for asymptomatic contacts of individuals with bubonic plague.

Infection Control: Use standard precautions for bubonic plague, and respiratory droplet precautions for suspected pneumonic plague. *Yersinia pestis* can survive in the environment for varying periods, but is susceptible to heat, disinfectants, and exposure to sunlight. Soap and water are effective if decontamination is needed.

OVERVIEW

Yersinia pestis is a rod-shaped, non-motile, non-sporulating, gram-negative bacterium of the family *Enterobacteraceae.* It causes plague, a zoonotic disease of rodents (e.g., rats, mice, ground squirrels). Humans typically develop disease through contact with infected rodents or, more commonly, their fleas. The biting fleas can transmit bacteria to humans, who then typically develop the bubonic form of plague. The bubonic form may progress to the septicemic and/or pneumonic forms. Larger outbreaks of human plague often follow epizootics in which large numbers of host rodents die off, leaving their fleas in search of other sources of a blood meal. Pneumonic plague would be the predominant form of disease expected after purposeful aerosol dissemination. All human populations are susceptible. Recovery from the disease is followed by temporary immunity. The organism remains viable in unchlorinated water, moist soil, and grains for several weeks. At near freezing temperatures, it will remain alive from months to years but is killed by 15 min of exposure to 55°C. It also remains viable for some time (hours to days) in dry sputum, flea feces, and buried bodies but is killed within several hours of exposure to sunlight.

HISTORY AND SIGNIFICANCE

Throughout recorded history, *Y. pestis* has been the cause of multiple human pandemics and countless deaths. Plague is now endemic worldwide yet is responsible for only sporadic human disease (200-4500 human cases including 30-200 deaths reported to the WHO annually). The United States worked with *Y. pestis* as a potential bioagent in the 1950s and 1960s before the old offensive biowarfare program was terminated. Other countries are suspected of having weaponized this organism. The Soviet Union had several institutes and thousands of scientists dedicated to identification, isolation, research and creating a biological weapon from Y. pestis. During World War II, Unit 731, of the Japanese Army, reportedly released plague-infected fleas from aircraft over Chinese cities. This method was cumbersome and unpredictable. The U.S. and Soviet Union developed the more reliable and effective delivery method of aerosolizing the organism.

The terrorist potential of plague was highlighted in 1995 when Larry Wayne Harris was arrested in Ohio for the illicit procurement of a *Y. pestis* culture through the mail. The contagious nature of pneumonic plague, whether through zoonotic or person-to-person transmission, makes it particularly concerning as a biological weapon.

CLINICAL FEATURES

Plague appears in three predominant forms in humans: bubonic, septicemic, and pneumonic. The vast majority of the 1 to 40 human cases reported annually in the U.S. are from the desert Southwest, where plague is endemic in rural rodent populations. Most naturally occurring human cases in the U.S. are bubonic (85%), with less primary septicemic (13%), or primary pneumonic (1-2%) disease.

Bubonic Plague. The bubonic form may occur after an infected flea bites a human host. The disease begins after a typical incubation period of 2-8 d, with acute and fulminant onset of nonspecific symptoms, including high fever (up to 40°C), severe malaise, headache, myalgias, and sometimes nausea and vomiting (25-50%). Up to half of patients will have abdominal pain. Simultaneous with, or shortly after, the onset of these nonspecific symptoms, the characteristic bubo develops – a swollen, extremely painful, infected lymph node. Buboes are typically 1-10 cm in diameter with erythema of the overlying skin and variable degrees of surrounding edema. They rarely become fluctuant or suppurate, and lymphangitis is uncommon. Buboes are most commonly seen in the femoral or inguinal lymph nodes as the legs are the most commonly flea-bitten part of the adult human body. But any lymph nodes can be involved, to include intra-abdominal nodes (presumably through hematogenous extension) which can present as a febrile patient with an acute abdomen. The liver and spleen are often tender and palpable. One quarter of patients will have some type of skin lesion: a pustule, vesicle, eschar or papule (containing leukocytes and bacteria) in the lymphatic drainage of the bubo, and presumably representing the site of the inoculating flea bite. Secondary septicemia is common, as greater than 80% of blood cultures are positive for the organism in patients with bubonic plague. However, only about a quarter of bubonic plague patients progress to clinical septicemia, typically within 2-6 d of symptom onset in untreated patients. In humans, the case fatality rate (CFR) of untreated bubonic plague is approximately 60%, but this is reduced to less than 5% with prompt, effective therapy.

Septicemic Plague. In those that do progress to secondary septicemia, as well as those presenting septicemic but without lymphadenopathy (primary septicemia), the symptoms and signs are similar to other gram-negative septicemias: high fever, chills, malaise, hypotension, tachycardia, tachypnea, nausea, vomiting, and diarrhea. All age groups can be affected, but the elderly seem to be at increased risk. Plague septicemia can produce thromboses in the acral vessels (presumably assisted by a low-temperature-activated coagulase protein produced by the organism), possibly leading to necrosis and gangrene, and disseminated intravascular coagulation (DIC); thus, black necrotic appendages may be accompanied by more proximal, purpuric lesions due to endotoxemia in advanced disease. Organisms can spread via the bloodstream to the lungs and, less commonly, to the CNS and elsewhere. Untreated septicemic plague is virtually 100% fatal, while treated disease carries a 30-50% mortality.

Pneumonic Plague. Pneumonic plague is an infection of the lungs due to either inhalation of the organisms (primary pneumonic plague), or spread to the lungs from septicemia (secondary pneumonic plague). Secondary pneumonic plague has been a complication in 12% of bubonic cases in the U.S. over the past 50 yrs. 28% of human plague cases resulting from exposure to plague-infected domestic cats in the US in recent decades presented as primary pneumonic plague; 25% of these human cases were in veterinarians or their assistants. Person-to-person spread of pneumonic plague has not occurred in the US since 1925. After an incubation period varying from 1 to 6 d for primary pneumonic plague (usually 2-4 d, and presumably dose-dependent), onset is acute and often fulminant. The first signs of illness include high fever, chills, headache, malaise, and myalgias, followed within 24 h by tachypnea and cough, eventually productive of bloody sputum. Although bloody sputum is characteristic, it can sometimes be watery or, less commonly, purulent. Gastrointestinal symptoms, including nausea, vomiting, diarrhea, and abdominal pain, may be present. Rarely, a cervical bubo might result from an inhalational exposure. CXR findings are variable, but most commonly reveal bilateral infiltrates, which may be patchy or consolidated. The pneumonia progresses rapidly, resulting in dyspnea, stridor, and cyanosis. The disease terminates with respiratory failure, and circulatory collapse. The CFR for pneumonic plague patients in the U.S. is approximately 50%. If untreated, the CFR for pneumonic plague is nearly 100%. In the U.S. in the past 50 yrs, 4 of the 7 pneumonic plague patients (57%) died. Recent data from the ongoing Madagascar epidemic, which began in 1989, corroborate that figure; the mortality associated with respiratory involvement was 57%, while that for bubonic plague was 15%.

Pneumonic plague is the only form of plague disease which readily spreads from person to person. From the sparse historical data available on past pneumonic plague epidemics, the average secondary infection rate is 1.3 cases per primary case (range 0 to 6). Transmission has been greatest under crowded, cold, and humid conditions. The majority of secondary cases have been in caregivers at home (80%) or medical professionals (14%) after close contact (within 6ft) with the primary cases.

Plague Meningitis. Meningitis is a rare complication of plague (up to 6 % of patients with septicemia, more common in children), most often occurring in bubonic or septicemic plague patients a week or more into illness. Typically these patients have been receiving sub-therapeutic doses of antibiotics or bacteriostatic antibiotics which do not cross the blood brain barrier well (e.g., tetracyclines). Signs and symptoms are consistent with subacute bacterial meningitis, and CSF demonstrates a leukocytosis with neutrophil predominance and perhaps gram-negative coccobacilli.

Nonspecific laboratory findings in all forms of plague disease include a leukocytosis, with a total WBC up to 20,000 cells per ml or more with increased band forms, and greater than 80% polymorphonuclear cells. Platelet counts can be normal or low. One also often finds increased fibrin split products and elevated partial thromboplastin time indicating a low-grade DIC. The blood urea nitrogen, creatinine, transaminases, and bilirubin may also be elevated, consistent with multiorgan failure.

DIAGNOSIS

Clinical diagnosis. Diagnosis of plague is based primarily on clinical suspicion. A patient with a painful bubo accompanied by fever, severe malaise and possible rodent exposure in an endemic area should raise suspicion of bubonic plague. The sudden appearance of large numbers of previously healthy patients with severe, rapidly progressive pneumonia with hemoptysis strongly suggests pneumonic plague as a result of an intentional aerosolization.

Laboratory diagnosis. A presumptive diagnosis can be made microscopically by identification of the coccobacillus in Gram (negative),

Wright, Giemsa, or Wayson's stains, or more specific immunofluorescence antibody-stained smears from lymph node needle aspirate, sputum, blood, or CSF samples. Bubo aspirates can be obtained by inserting a 20 gauge needle on a 10 ml syringe containing 1ml of sterile saline; saline is injected and withdrawn until blood tinged. Definitive diagnosis relies on culturing the organism from clinical specimens. The organism grows slowly at normal incubation temperatures (optimal growth at 25-28°C), and may be misidentified by automated systems (often as *Y. pseudotuberculosis)* because of delayed biochemical reactions. It may be cultured on blood agar, MacConkey agar, or infusion broth. It will also grow in automated culture systems. Any patient with suspected plague should have blood cultures performed; as bacteremia can be intermittent, multiple cultures should be obtained, preferably before receipt of antibiotics (clinical severity permitting). Confirmatory diagnosis via culture commonly takes 48-72 h (cultures should be held for 5-7 d); thus specific antibiotic therapy for plague must not be withheld pending culture results. Confirmatory culture-based diagnosis is made by specific bacteriophage lysis of the organism, which is available at reference laboratories.

Most naturally occurring strains of *Y. pestis* produce an F1-antigen in vivo, which can be detected in serum samples by specific immunoassay. A single anti-F1 titer of >1:10 by agglutination testing is suggestive of plague, while a single titer of >1:128 in a patient who has not previously been exposed to plague or received a plague vaccine is more specific; a fourfold rise in acute vs. convalescent antibody titers in patient serum is probably the most specific serologic method to confirm diagnosis, but results are available only retrospectively. Most patients will seroconvert within 1-2 wks of disease onset, but a minority require 3 or more wks.

PCR (using specific primers), is not sufficiently developed yet for routine use, but it is a very sensitive and specific technique, currently able to identify as few as 10 organisms per ml.

Most clinical assays can be performed in BSL-2 laboratories, whereas procedures producing aerosols or yielding significant quantities of organisms require BSL-3 containment.

MEDICAL MANAGEMENT

Antibiotics. Prompt initiation of appropriate antibiotics is paramount for reducing mortality; this is especially true in primary pneumonic plague, for which CFRs approach 100% if adequate therapy is not initiated within 18-24 h of onset of symptoms. Initial empiric therapy for systemic disease caused by *Y. pestis* includes at least one of the following antibiotics.

Preferred

- **Streptomycin** (FDA approved),* 1g IM bid (15 mg/kg IM bid for children (up to 2 gm/d)), or
- **Gentamicin** 5 mg/kg IM or IV qd, or 2 mg/kg loading dose followed by 1.7 mg/kg IM or IV q 8 h (2.5 mg/kg IV q 8 hr for children),(adjusted for renal clearance), or

Alternatives

- Doxycycline (FDA approved), 100 mg IV q12 h or 200mg IV qd for adults or children ≥ 45 kg (2.2 mg/kg IV q 12 h for children <45 kg), or
- Ciprofloxacin 400 mg IV every 12 h for adults (for children use 15 mg/kg IV q 12 h (up to 1 gm/d)), or
- Chloramphenicol, 25 mg/kg IV, then 15 mg/kg IV q 6 h (adjusted for serum levels, and not for children less than 2 yrs old)

IV antibiotics can be switched to oral as the improvement in the patient's clinical course dictates, to complete at least 10-14 total d of therapy. For treatment of plague meningitis, add IV chloramphenicol. Patients with uncomplicated bubonic plague often demonstrate resolution of fever and other systemic symptoms within 3-5 d, while more complicated bubonic disease, septicemic, and pneumonic plague often result in extended hospital courses.

It is imperative that antibiotics are adjusted for demonstrated susceptibility patterns for the infecting strain; naturally occurring strains have been reported which are resistant to streptomycin, tetracyclines, and chloramphenocol, and it is anticipated that weaponized plague could be intentionally rendered antibiotic resistant. Despite typically good in vitro susceptibilities to penicillins and cephalosporins, these antibiotics are generally felt to be ineffective in treating plague; in fact, animal studies

---

*Streptomycin has historically been the drug of choice for plague and is the only aminoglycoside antibiotic approved by the FDA for treatment of plague; however, because it may not be readily available immediately after a large-scale biowarfare attack, gentamicin and other alternative drugs should be considered first.

suggest that beta-lactam antibiotics may accelerate mortality in bacteremic mice. Macrolide antibiotics are ineffective for plague.

Supportive therapy includes IV crystalloids and hemodynamic monitoring. Although low-grade DIC may occur, clinically significant hemorrhage is uncommon, as is the need to treat with heparin. Endotoxic shock is common, but pressor agents are rarely needed. Finally, buboes rarely require any form of local care, but instead recede with systemic antibiotic therapy. In fact, incision and drainage poses an infection risk to others in contact with the patient due to aerosolization of the bubo contents. Needle aspiration is recommended for diagnostic purposes and may provide symptomatic relief.

Infection Control. Use standard precautions for bubonic and septicemic plague patients. Suspected pneumonic plague cases require strict isolation with respiratory droplet precautions for at least 48 h after initiation of antibiotic therapy, or until sputum cultures are negative in confirmed cases. Historically, epidemics of pneumonic plague have subsided rapidly with implementation of such relatively simple infection control measures. Pneumonic plague patients being transported should wear a surgical mask when feasible. If competent vectors (fleas) and reservoirs (rodents) are present, measures must be taken to prevent local disease cycles. These might include: use of flea insecticides, rodent control measures (after or during flea control), and flea barriers for patient-care areas.

PROPHYLAXIS

Vaccine. No vaccine is currently available for prophylaxis of plague. A licensed, killed whole-cell vaccine was available in the U.S. from 1946 until November 1998. It offered protection against bubonic plague, but was not effective against aerosolized *Y. pestis*. The plague bacterium secretes several virulence factors which as subunit proteins are immunogenic and possess protective properties. Among these has been Fraction 1 (F1) and V (virulence) proteins. As combined recombinants (fusion) proteins, these products have been the focus of plague vaccine development and have shown promise in preclinical and phase 1 and phase 2 clinical trials. Recently, an F1-V antigen (fusion protein) vaccine developed at USAMRIID protected mice for a year against an inhalational challenge.

Immunoprophylaxis. There is no passive immunoprophylaxis (i.e., immune globulin) available for pre- or postexposure management of plague.

Preexposure chemoprophylaxis: No antibiotics are licensed by the FDA for use before exposure to plague. However, chemoprophylaxis with doxycycline (or ciprofloxacin) may protect against plague based upon in vitro susceptibilities.

Postexposure chemoprophylaxis: Face-to-face contacts (within 2 meters) of patients with pneumonic plague or persons possibly exposed to a plague aerosol (i.e., in a biowarfare attack) should be given antibiotic prophylaxis for 7 d or the duration of risk of exposure plus 7 d. If fever or cough occurs in these individuals, a full treatment course with antibiotics should be started.

Preferred empiric prophylaxis

- Doxycycline 100 mg PO bid for adults and children ≥45 kg (for children <45 kg use 2.2 mg / kg PO bid), or

Alternatives

- Ciprofloxacin 500 mg PO bid for adults (20 mg/kg PO bid (up to 1 gm/d) for children)
- Chloramphenicol, 25 mg/kg PO qid

Other tetracyclines and fluoroquinolones could potentially be substituted for doxycycline and ciprofloxacin, respectively. TMP/SMX may represent a second-line alternative, should susceptibilities allow. Chemoprophylaxis is generally not recommended after contact with bubonic or septicemic plague patients; however, individuals making such contacts, especially if sharing the same environment in which the patient received a natural exposure, should be observed for symptoms for a week. If symptoms occur, start treatment antibiotics while awaiting results of diagnostic studies.

Q-Fever

SUMMARY

Signs and Symptoms: Q-fever manifests in two disease forms: acute and chronic. Some authorities now consider the long-term sequelae that may develop to be a third. Route and magnitude of exposure largely determine the disease manifestation that develops -- e.g., pneumonia follows an aerosol exposure. Up to 60% of human infections are inapparent. In the remaining 40% of clinical cases, a non-specific flu-like illness predominates with a minority of individuals developing immunosuppression, fever, headaches, pneumonia or hepatitis. Incubation period is estimated at 1 to 5 weeks (10 to 17 days in one study) and the duration of symptoms ranges from a few days to a few months. Chronic disease may manifest many months or years after the primary infection, with the most frequent and serious presentation being endocarditis, which is usually fatal if not treated. Most recently, a chronic fatigue syndrome has been identified as a possible sequela.

Diagnosis: The combination of frequent subclinical disease, sporadic local occurrence and non-specific signs and symptoms makes Q-fever diagnosis problematic. Careful history may reveal risk factors (working around livestock, travelling in endemic areas) and raise suspicion, but definitive diagnosis requires serological testing (indirect fluorescent antibody, complement fixation, ELISA), PCR, or *Coxiella burnetii* positive blood or tissue cultures (requires BSL-3 facilities).

Treatment: Most cases will resolve without therapy, but it is generally accepted that all acute patients should receive antimicrobials. Oral tetracycline (500 mg q6h) or doxycycline (100 mg q12h) are the treatments of choice and should be administered for 7 to 14 days, or at least 3 days post fever remission. For acute patients with pre-existing disease, such as valvulopathy, 12 to 18 months of doxy may be necessary. Chronic Q-fever may require years, or in some cases lifetime, therapy, but a combination of doxy (100mg q12h) and hydroxychloroquine (200mg q8h) for 18 months may be sufficient. Other drugs that can penetrate and are active in the eukaryotic cell, such as the quinolones and newer macrolides, may be suitable alternative therapies.

Prophylaxis: Antimicrobials appear to be the most effective if begun within the first 3 days of illness. For prophylaxis in suspected exposures, doxy given at 8 to12 days post exposure (but not before) appears to be effective. A licensed vaccine (Q-Vax) is available in Australia and Europe. In the U.S., work continues on a vaccine for use in individuals at high-risk. Pre-vaccination screening is essential as those who were previously exposed to Q-fever, or to a Q-fever vaccine, may develop severe local or systemic disease following vaccination.

Isolation and Decontamination: Standard precautions are recommended for healthcare workers dealing with suspected or confirmed cases. For autopsies, precautions should be taken to prevent aerosolization of body fluids. If culturing of the organism is to be performed, it must be done in a BSL-3 facility. Q-fever is primarily considered to be a zoonotic disease, with human-to-human, or tick-to-human transmission being very rare. The spore form of the organism is very hardy and can survive for years in the environment. It can probably survive direct UV radiation, dilute bleach and typical disinfectants. Autoclaving and boiling for 10 min will kill the organism. Decontamination may be attempted with a 1:100 *Lysol* solution, 1 % sodium hypochlorite solution, 5 % hydrogen peroxide, or 70% ethanol. The M291 skin decontamination kit will not neutralize the organism.

OVERVIEW

Q-fever is a zoonotic (transmitted from animal to man) disease caused by the obligate intracellular, gram-negative bacterium *Coxiella burnetii*. Q-fever is found world-wide, with the exception of New Zealand. Its natural reservoirs are numerous and include sheep, cattle, goats, rabbits, cats, dogs, rodents, birds and ticks. The organism localizes in the gravid uterus and mammary glands of infected animals and is shed in very high numbers at parturition, whether at or before term. Transmission to humans is typically via aerosolization of infectious particles, especially in premises contaminated with fetal membranes, birth fluids, aborted fetuses, and excreta from infected animals in locations where infected animals and their by-products are processed, as well as at necropsy sites. Infection in livestock occasionally results in abortion, stillbirth, and dystocia, but is often asymptomatic. Transmission may also occur by ingesting contaminated raw milk and cheese, through blood product transfusions, vertically (mother to offspring), and by tick vectors. Tick bites are believed to be important in maintaining disease in livestock and wild animal reservoirs, but is less important in human disease. *C. burnetii* may be found in high numbers in tick feces with consequent environmental contamination. Viable organisms have been isolated from bull semen and sexual transmission is believed to be possible in humans.

The infectious dose is extremely low; a single bacterium may lead to infection in 50% of people (ID_{50}). Concentrations of the organism in a gram of placental tissue may be as high as 10^9 per gram. Infected livestock, even if asymptomatic, shed large numbers of organisms in placental tissues and body fluids including milk, urine, and feces. Direct exposure to these, or to sites contaminated by them, is a significant risk factor. Humans acquire Q-fever primarily by inhaling the aerosolized organism. Farmers, abattoir workers, and hunters are at greatest risk for exposure. *C. burnetii* is also a significant hazard in laboratory personnel who are working with the organism.

Q-fever is endemic to many areas and natural outbreaks occur regularly. From 2007 through late 2010, almost 3,500 human cases were reported in an on-going, natural outbreak in the Netherlands which included 6 deaths. The long-term socio-economic consequences of this particular outbreak are not yet apparent.

HISTORY AND SIGNIFICANCE

Q-fever was first described in 1935 in Brisbane, Australia, by Edward Holbrook Derrick after an outbreak of febrile illness among abattoir workers. It was called "Query fever" because the causative agent was initially unknown. No diagnosis could be made based on the varied patient histories, physical exam findings and investigations. Australian researchers Frank Macfarlane Burnet and Mavis Freeman (1937) identified a fastidious, intracellular bacterium in guinea pigs that had been injected with body fluids from Derrick's patients. Almost at the same time, in the U.S., a rickettsia-like bacterium was isolated from ticks by Herald Cox. These agents were later determined to be identical. Burnet was first to isolate and describe the organism in 1937, and Cox described vector transmission from ticks in 1938. The bacterium was named *Coxiella burnetii* to honor these researchers.

C. burnetii is classified as a Category B pathogen. Very large numbers of bacteria can be produced and the spore form, being resistant to many environmental factors and stable for years, makes it highly suitable for aerosol delivery. Even with low mortality and moderate morbidity rates, the number of individuals seeking treatment (required or not) could be immense.

CLINICAL FEATURES

As Derrick discovered when attempting diagnose the original patients, it is really not possible to describe a "normal" clinical presentation of the disease. A health care provider will likely be forced to make a presumptive diagnosis that includes Q-fever as a "rule out". With varying incubation periods and a vague flu-like illness being the most common presentation in acute cases, a clinical diagnosis will be impossible. For naturally occurring outbreaks, in which human numbers are typically low (the recent Netherland's outbreak mentioned earlier being an exception), the majority of cases may go undiagnosed. (Remember that 60% of individuals will be asymptomatic.) Approximately of outbreak victims have been male, with a preponderance in those over 15 years of age. With the intentional release of large numbers of bacteria, there may be more uniformity in the clinical presentations, as there is expected to be some correlation between the severity and physical manifestation of disease to this route and magnitude of exposure.

Acute Q-fever: Historically, up to 60% of acute infections have shown no clinical sign of disease. This may not hold true in an intentional release, as the exposure levels are potentially much higher. In natural outbreaks, 40% develop a non-specific flu-like illness, that can include severe headache, joint and/or muscle pain, fever (which may last for months in untreated patients, otherwise reaching a peak of 102-105° F degrees after 3 days, then returning abruptly to normal after 5 to 14 days in treated individuals) and cough (often productive). This may be accompanied by varying emergence of atypical pneumonia (with or without pleural effusion) and hepatitis (with ALP, ALT and AST reaching 2-3X ULN). Around 2% of cases will develop myocarditis (pericarditis and pericardial effusion), which is the leading cause of death in acute Q-fever patients. Up to 20% will develop a skin rash. Weight loss may occur. There appears to be a geographic distribution to which symptom predominates. A host of other disease states have been linked to acute Q-fever, including various neurological disorders (especially with cranial nerve involvement), gastroenteritis, orchitis, lymphadenopathy and bone–marrow necrosis. It is recommended that all acute Q-fever patients have an echocardiogram. Abortion occurs in 100% of women if infection occurs during the first trimester of pregnancy.

Chronic Q-fever: Chronic Q-fever is rare (< 10% of cases), but is potentially a much more serious condition than the acute form. It may not manifest for up to 20 years. Individuals with pre-existing heart disease (especially cardiac valve disease) are pre-disposed to developing endocarditis. Chronic Q-fever may also result in abortion, premature birth, or low birth weight, if the disease recrudesces during pregnancy.

DIAGNOSIS

The relatively vague nature of the symptoms means that the Q-fever differential diagnosis is quite extensive. A characteristic pattern of cases associated with a geographic area or compressed time period should raise suspicion. For Warfighters, other bio-agents that have overlapping symptoms should be considered (e.g., plague, anthrax and tularemia pneumonias) in addition to Q-fever. Definitive diagnosis requires laboratory testing.

Culture: Any potential amplification of *C. burnetii* must be performed in a BSL-3 facility, as the risk of aerosolization is great and considering the highly infective nature of *C. burnetii* (ID_{50} of 1), biological containment and special handling are essential. Standard plate or liquid media will not support the growth of *C. burnetii*, as the bacterium is an obligate intracellular organism and requires mammalian cells to replicate. Bacterial isolation and amplification may be carried out using HEL cells and Shell Vial centrifugation. More recently, a cell-free method for *C. burnetii* growth was developed using defined media and atmospheric conditions (Omsland, *et al*, 2009). Isolating the bacterium from tissue samples is considered the gold standard for identification, but the process lacks sensitivity. More often, serological methods will allow for the identification of etiologic agent and status of disease.

Serology: Indirect immunofluorescence is the current reference method for diagnosis of Q-fever. Enzyme immunoassay, autoimmunohistochemistry and complement fixation are also being used to diagnose Q-fever. PCR detection (conventional, Light-Cycler Nested and real time) allows for rapid, sensitive and specific detection of *C. burnetii* origin DNA in samples ranging from serum to tissue biopsies. As there are usually bacteria present in the serum in acute infection, PCR allows for detection well before serum antibodies against Q-fever are present. Serum antibody detection, in addition to allowing for disease identification may be useful in determining if the disease is acute or chronic. Specific IgM antibodies against phase II antigen may be detectable as early as the second week after onset of illness and remain elevated for up to 3 months. Combined detection of IgM, IgA, and IgG antibodies improves assay specificity and provides accuracy in diagnosis. Two antigenic phases of *C. burnetii* infections exist: phase I (virulent) and phase II (avirulent). Acute Q-fever cases usually exhibit a much higher antibody level to phase II (first detected during the second week of illness). Antibodies to phase I antigens of *C. burnetii* generally take longer to appear and indicate continued exposure to bacteria. High levels of antibody to phase I in later isolates in conjunction with constant or falling levels of antibody to phase II suggest chronic Q-fever (Table 1). Antibodies to phase I and II antigens may persist for months or years after initial infection. Seroconversion, or a fourfold rise in titer (requires a baseline and repeat testing in 2 to 4 weeks) indicates an acute infection. Elevated IgG of greater than 1:200 and IgM greater than 1:25 to phase II also supports an acute infection. In chronic disease states, a 1:800 IgG or greater than 1:59 IgA against phase I antigen suggest a chronic infection exists. ELISA is available at USAMRIID in which a single serum specimen can be used to reliably diagnose acute Q-fever as early as 10 to 14 days into illness.

TABLE 1. **Antibodies generally present during acute and chronic Q-fever infection**

	IgA Antibody Phase		IgM Antibody Phase		IgG Antibody Phase	
Infection Stage	I	II	I	II	I	II
Acute			X	X		X
Chronic	X				X	

Blood Chemistry and Complete Blood Counts: A CBC is usually unremarkable excepting leukocytosis (14 to 21×10^9/L) in about 25%. Thrombocytopenia may also be seen in up to a third of patients in the acute phase, with thrombcytosis developing during the recovery phase. Erythrocyte sedimentation rate (ESR) typically is mildly elevated. Liver function tests in up to 85 % of patients show a 2- or 3-fold elevation in ALP and the transaminases (AST, ALT). Bilirubin is usually normal. Hepatitis patients and those with chronic Q-fever frequently have circulating autoantibodies, including anti-smooth muscle, anti-cardiolipin, anti-phospholipid, anti-clotting factor (thus liver biopsy may risk hemorrhage), and antinuclear antibodies. Endocarditis usually causes a significantly elevated ESR, often with anemia, thrombocytopenia, and polyclonal hypergammaglobulinemia.

Blood cultures on standard media are invariably negative, as *C. burnetii* will only grow in living cells or organisms; even so, most labs do not attempt cell culture as it poses a significant infection risk to laboratory personnel (BSL-3 precautions) and is often less sensitive than serology. Sputum examination is unremarkable even in patients with productive cough. Mild lymphocytic pleocytosis is common in the CSF of patients with meningoencephalitis. Liver biopsy in hepatitis patients or bone biopsy in patients with osteomyelitis may reveal granulomas.

Imaging Studies: Findings on CXR are non-specific and may be normal in up to 10% of those with acute Q-fever. Pleural effusions are rare. Sonography may reveal granulomatous lesions, particularly of the liver, even in asymptomatic patients. This may be accompanied by palpation of a mass in the right hypochondrium. Pericardial effusion may suggest pericarditis and/or myocarditis. Transesophageal echocardiography is more sensitive in finding the typically small and subendothelial lesions of endocarditis. A thorough echocardiogram may help identify non-symptomatic heart disease that could pre-dispose individuals to develop chronic Q-fever. Chronic disease findings include cardiac valve abnormalities (vegetation, regurgitation, abscess) and granulomatous hepatitis.

MEDICAL MANAGEMENT

Standard precautions are recommended for healthcare workers dealing with suspected or confirmed cases of Q-fever. For autopsies, or when handling surgical or tissue biopsies, precautions should be taken to prevent aerosolization of body fluids. Autoclaving and boiling for 10 min will kill the organism in samples no longer needed. Decontamination may be attempted with a 1:100 *Lysol* solution, 1 % sodium hypochlorite solution, 5% hydrogen peroxide, or 70% ethanol. The M291 skin decontamination kit will not neutralize the organism.

Acute Q-fever

Adults: Doxycycline 100 mg q12 hrs, with or without hydroxychloroquine (which alkalinizes the phagolysosomes and may make doxy bactericidal) for at least 14 days is the treatment of choice for acute Q-fever. Tetracycline 500 mg q 6 hrs could be used as an alternative. Antibiotics are most effective if begun within 3 days of the onset of symptoms. Fever usually disappears within 3 or 4 days after treatment is begun. Relapse is not uncommon and may be associated with an antibiotic regimen discontinued within 2 weeks. Ciprofloxacin and other quinolones are active *in vitro* and should be considered in patients unable to take tetracycline or doxy, but they may require longer courses (14 to 21 days) to be effective. Quinolones may be a better choice than tetracyclines for patients with meningoencephalitis as they penetrate the CSF more consistently. Trimethoprim-sulfamethoxazole (TMP-SMX) or macrolides (especially newer macrolides like clarithromycin or azithromycin) may represent alternative therapies for patients for whom doxy or quinolones are contraindicated.

Children: Ideal therapy for acute Q-fever in children less than 8 years old (for whom doxy is contraindicated) has not been determined; some clinicians recommend TMP-SMX for this group, while macrolides may be useful alternatives.

Chronic Q-fever

Successful treatment of Q-fever endocarditis is difficult. Combination therapy of doxy with quinolones for at least 3 to 4 years, or doxy 100 mg q 12 hrs, with hydroxychloroquine 200 mg q 8 hrs for at least 18 months is recommended. The latter regimen leads to fewer relapses; however, it requires routine eye examination to monitor for hydroxychloroquine-associated ocular toxicity or visual field changes. Valve replacement may be required to cure Q-fever endocarditis. Women who have contracted acute Q-fever during pregnancy should have specific serum antibody titers determined postpartum; those with evidence of chronic Q-fever by serology are often treated with at least 12 months of doxy plus hydroxychloroquine. For all forms of chronic Q-fever specific serum antibody titers are followed (typically every

3 months); antibiotics should be continued until phase I *C. burnetii* IgG and IgA levels drop to 1:200 or less.

Long term sequelae: A chronic fatigue syndrome has been reported as a possible long term complication following acute Q-fever infection. The condition may include fatigue, muscle and joint pain, night sweats and behavioral changes (mood and sleep patterns) and may strike up to 20% of those with a history of acute infection. Treatment for this disorder is largely symptomatic and may require a combination of physical and pharmacological intervention.

PROPHYLAXIS

Vaccine: A licensed Q-fever vaccine is available in Australia and Eastern Europe. Administration in already immune or pre-sensitized individuals may cause severe local induration, sterile abscess formation, and necrosis at the inoculation site and thus absence of prior exposure must first be determined. This is accomplished by an intradermal skin test using 0.02 mg of vaccine. Vaccination with a single dose of this killed suspension of *C. burnetii* provides complete protection against naturally occurring Q-fever, and greater than 95% protection against aerosol exposure. Protection lasts for at least 5 years. A formalin-inactivated whole cell IND vaccine is available for vaccinating at-risk personnel on an investigational basis has been available in the U.S.

Antibiotics: Chemoprophylaxis begun 8 to 12 days post-exposure is effective, with tetracycline 500 mg q 6 hrs or doxy 100 mg q 12 hrs for at least 5 to 7 days. Chemoprophylaxis given within 1 to 7 days of exposure is not effective and may only prolong the onset of disease.

CONTROL

As with many zoonotic outbreaks, investigations are done in cooperation with animal health authorities to determine whether the source is naturally occurring or the result of an intentional release. Animal health authorities can also help to control outbreaks that may be propagated by intentionally or unintentionally infected livestock sources, and ensure that dairy products are pasteurized and from approved sources.

Tularemia

SUMMARY

Signs and Symptoms: Historically, tularemia has manifested as either ulceroglandular or typhoidal. Ulceroglandular tularemia presents with a local ulcer and regional lymphadenopathy, fever, chills, headache, and malaise. Typhoidal tularemia presents with fever, headache, malaise, prostration, and often substernal discomfort and a non-productive cough. Other clinical forms are known to exist.

Diagnosis: CXR may reveal a pneumonic process, mediastinal or hilar lymphadenopathy, or pleural effusion. Routine culture (blood, sputum, ulcers and/or pharyngeal sites) is possible but difficult. The diagnosis can be established retrospectively by serology. Presumptive tests include direct fluorescence antibody and PCR.

Treatment: Administration of antibiotics (streptomycin or gentamicin) with early treatment is very effective for naturally acquired disease.

Prophylaxis: A live, attenuated vaccine is available as an IND. It is administered as a one-time dose by scarification. A 2 wk course of doxycycline or ciprofloxacin should be effective as prophylaxis when given after exposure to a susceptible strain.

Isolation and Decontamination: Standard precautions for healthcare workers. Organisms are relatively easy to render harmless by mild heat (55° C for 10 min) and standard disinfectants.

OVERVIEW

Francisella tularensis, the causative agent of tularemia, is a small, aerobic non-motile, gram-negative coccobacillus. Tularemia (also known as rabbit fever and deer fly fever) is a zoonotic disease that humans typically acquire after skin or mucous membranes contact with tissues or body fluids of infected animals, or from bites of infected arthropods such as ticks, deerflies, or mosquitoes. Less commonly, inhaling contaminated aerosols or ingesting contaminated foods or water may produce clinical disease. Respiratory exposure to infectious aerosols would typically cause typhoidal tularemia with pneumonia, but rarely ulceroglandular or oculoglandular forms can be seen as well. The organism is found throughout the temperate northern hemisphere and is typically the cause of only sporadic human disease (approximately 125 cases per year in the U.S. from 2000-2008), but is infrequently the cause of large human epidemics associated with animal epizootics. *F. tularensis* exists in at least two variants, or biovars: Biovar A, which is the predominant causes of human disease in North America; and Biovar B, a less virulent form which predominates in northern Europe and Asia. The organism can remain viable for weeks in water, soil, carcasses, hides, and for years in frozen rabbit meat. It is resistant for months to temperatures of freezing and below. It is easily killed by heat and disinfectants.

HISTORY AND SIGNIFICANCE

F. tularensis was identified as a distinct organism in 1911 during an investigation of a plague-like disease in ground squirrels in Tulare County, California. A US Public Health Service physician, Edward Francis, established the cause of the "deer-fly fever" as *Bacterium tularense* and subsequently devoted his life to researching the organism and disease, hence, the organism was later renamed *Francisella tularensis*. *F. tularensis* has been responsible for large waterborne epidemics. During the German siege of Stalingrad in WWII, there were perhaps hundreds of thousands of human cases, many of which were pulmonary, leading to speculation that this may have resulted from the intentional use of tularemia as a biological weapon. However, there was also an ongoing and concurrent epizootic in rodents and thousands of human cases were documented in the area before the siege. This suggests a natural cause for this epidemic. In Sweden during the winter of 1966-67, hundreds of cases, most of which were pulmonary, occurred in farmers who processed hay contaminated by infected rodents.

F. tularensis was weaponized by the U.S. in the 1950s and 1960s during the offensive biowarfare program. Other countries are suspected to have weaponized this agent as well. This organism can be stabilized to create an offensive weapon by an adversary similar to the other bacterial agents discussed in this handbook.

CLINICAL FEATURES

After an incubation period of 3-6 d (range 1-21 d; likely dose dependent), onset is usually acute. Tularemia may appear in any of several forms, which can generally be categorized as either typhoidal or ulceroglandular. In humans, as few as 10 organisms will cause disease if injected intradermally, 10-50 organisms cause illness via inhalation, whereas approximately 10^8 organisms are required with oral challenge.

Typhoidal tularemia (5-15% of naturally acquired cases) occurs mainly after inhalation of infectious aerosols but can occur after intradermal or gastrointestinal challenge. The disease manifests as a nonspecific syndrome consisting of abrupt onset of fever (38-40°C), headache, malaise, myalgias, and prostration; but unlike most other forms of tularemia disease, it presents without lymphadenopathy. Occasionally patients will present with nausea, vomiting, diarrhea, or abdominal pain. Case fatality rates (CFRs) are approximately 35% in untreated, naturally acquired typhoidal cases. Survivors of untreated tularemia may have symptoms which persist for weeks or, less often, months, with progressive debilitation. Mortality is higher if pneumonia is also present; this is the form of disease most likely to be seen after an aerosol biowarfare attack. CFRs after a biowarfare attack may be greater than the 1-3% seen with appropriately treated natural disease.

Ulceroglandular tularemia (75-85% of naturally acquired cases) is most often acquired through inoculation of the skin or mucous membranes with blood or tissue fluids of infected animals. It is usually characterized by usually sudden onset of fever (85%), chills (52%), headache (45%), cough (38%), and myalgias (31%), concurrent with the appearance of a painful papule at the site of inoculation. The papule progresses rapidly to pustule, then a painful ulcer, accompanied by development of painful regional lymphadenopathy. Cutaneous ulcers are generally 0.4 to 3.0 cm in diameter with heaped edges. Lymph nodes are 0.5 to 10 cm in diameter and usually tender. In 5-10% of cases there is focal lymphadenopathy without an obvious ulcer present. Enlarged nodes can become fluctuant and spontaneously drain even when the patient has been taking antibiotics, and, if untreated, can persist for months or even years.

In a minority of cases (1-2%) the site of primary inoculation is in the eye (oculoglandular disease); this occurs after inoculation of the conjunctivae by contaminated hands, by splattering of infected tissue fluids, or via infectious aerosols. Patients have unilateral, painful, purulent conjunctivitis with preauricular or cervical lymphadenopathy. Chemosis, periorbital edema, and small nodular granulomatous lesions or ulcerations of the conjunctiva are noted in some patients.

Pharyngitis can occur in up to 25% of all patients with tularemia. It usually presents as an acute exudative pharyngitis or tonsillitis, sometimes with ulceration and associated painful cervical lymphadenopathy. It may occur as a syndrome of isolated penicillin-unresponsive pharyngitis and mistaken for infectious mononucleosis or other viral pharyngitis.

Pulmonary involvement is present in 47-94% of all naturally occurring cases of tularemia. It may be severe and fulminant or mild and asymptomatic and can be associated with any form of tularemia (seen in 30% of ulceroglandular cases), but it is most common in typhoidal tularemia (up to 80% of cases). Pneumonitis is asymptomatic in up to 30% of cases but more commonly presents with non-productive cough and substernal chest pain and occasionally with pleuritic chest pain, dyspnea, purulent sputum, or hemoptysis. An atypical or interstitial perihilar process is common but fulminant lobar pneumonias, bronchiolitis, cavitary lesions, bronchopleural fistulas, and chronic, granulomatous processes have all been described. Hilar adenopathy is common and pleural effusions have been recorded in 15% of cases. Thirty percent of cases of tularemia pneumonia may be accompanied by pharyngitis. Like pneumonic plague, tularemia pneumonia can be primary after the inhalation of organisms or secondary after hematogenous spread from other sites. Untreated, CFRs can approach 60%.

DIAGNOSIS

Clinical diagnosis. A clue to the diagnosis of tularemia after a biowarfare attack with *F. tularensis* might be a large number of temporally clustered patients presenting with similar nonspecific, febrile, systemic illnesses progressing rapidly to life-threatening pleuropneumonitis. Differential diagnoses include typhoidal syndromes (e.g., typhoid fever, rickettsia, or malaria) or pneumonic processes (e.g., plague, mycoplasma, influenza, Q-fever, staphylococcal enterotoxin B). Even after an aerosol biowarfare attack, a percentage of patients should be expected to present with ulceroglandular disease. Some patients may exhibit a pulse-temperature mismatch (seen as often as 40% of the time in naturally acquired disease). The systemic symptoms and signs (e.g., fever) of tularemia classically respond quickly to appropriate antibiotics; patients typically improve dramatically within 24-48 h of initiation of aminoglycosides (e.g., streptomycin or gentamicin), tetracyclines (e.g. doxycycline), or fluoroquinolones (e.g., ciprofloxacin). In contrast patients may remain febrile for weeks while on penicillin or cephalosporins alone.

Radiologic diagnosis. CXR should be performed if systemic tularemia disease is suspected, but findings are often nonspecific. Atypical pneumonia accompanied by hilar adenopathy or other pulmonary findings on CXR in the absence of clinical findings of pulmonary disease, could be clues to tularemia in some cases.

Laboratory diagnosis. Initial laboratory evaluations are generally nonspecific. Peripheral WBC counts usually range from 5,000 to 22,000 cells per microliter. Differential blood cell counts are normal with occasional lymphocytosis late in the disease process. Hematocrit, hemoglobin, and platelet levels are usually normal. Mild elevations in lactose dehydrogenase, serum transaminases, and alkaline phosphatase are common. Rhabdomyolysis may be associated with elevations in serum creatine kinase and urinary myoglobin levels. CSF is usually normal, although mild abnormalities in protein, glucose, and blood cell counts have been reported.

Tularemia can be diagnosed by recovering the organism in culture from blood, ulcers, conjunctival exudates, sputum, gastric washings, and pharyngeal exudates. Recovery of organisms may even be possible after the institution of appropriate antibiotic therapy. However, unless tularemia is suspected, delays in diagnosis are probable as the organism does not grow well in standard clinical laboratory media. *F. tularensis* produces small, smooth, opaque colonies after 48 to 72 h on medium containing cysteine or other sulfhydryl compounds (e.g., glucose cysteine blood agar, thioglycollate broth). Isolation represents a clear hazard to laboratory personnel and culture should only be attempted in BSL-3 containment.

Most diagnoses of tularemia are made serologically using bacterial agglutination or ELISA. Antibodies to *F. tularensis* appear within the first week of infection but levels adequate to allow confidence in the specificity of the serologic diagnosis (titer > 1:160) do not appear until more than 2 wks after infection. Because cross-reactions can occur with *Brucella* spp., *Proteus* OX19, and *Yersinia* organisms and because antibodies may persist for years after infection, diagnosis should be made only if a fourfold or greater increase in the tularemia tube agglutination or microagglutination titer is seen during the course of the illness. Titers are usually negative the first week of infection, positive the second week in 50-70% of cases, and reach a maximum in 4-8 wks.

MEDICAL MANAGEMENT

Treatment. Initial empiric therapy for systemic disease caused by *F. tularensis* includes at least one of the following antibiotics.

Preferred

- **Streptomycin,*** 1g IM bid (15 mg/kg IM bid for children), or
- **Gentamicin** 5 mg/kg IM or IV qd (2.5 mg/kg IM or IV q8 hr for children), or

Alternatives

- **Doxycycline**, 100 mg IV q12 h for adults or children 45 kg (2.2 mg/kg IV q12 h for children < 45 kg), or
- **Ciprofloxacin** 400 mg IV every 12 h for adults (for children use 15 mg/g IV q12 h (up to 1 gm/d)), or
- **Chloramphenicol**, 15 mg/kg IV q6 h

IV antibiotics can be switched to oral as the improvement in the patient's course dictates. Length of therapy depends upon the antibiotic used. Chloramphenicol and tetracyclines (doxycycline) have been associated with relapse with courses lasting even 2 wks and thus should be continued for at least 14 to 21 d. Streptomycin, gentamicin, and ciprofloxacin should be continued for at least 10 to 14 d. It is quite possible that any intentional use of tularemia as a weapon will employ a strain of the organism which is resistant to our preferred antibiotics. Thus testing the strain for antibiotic susceptibilities is of paramount importance. A clinical clue to resistance would be failure of the patient to improve dramatically after 24 to 48 h of antibiotics.

Infection Control. As there is no known human-to-human transmission of tularemia, neither isolation nor quarantine is necessary. Standard precautions are appropriate for care of patients with draining lesions or pneumonia. Strict adherence to the drainage / secretion recommendations of standard precautions is required, especially for draining lesions, and for the disinfection of soiled clothing, bedding, equipment, etc. Heat and

*Streptomycin his historically been the drug of choice for tularemia and is the only aminoglycoside antibiotic approved by the FDA for treatment of tularemia; however, because it may not be readily available immediately after a large-scale biowarfare attack, gentamicin and other alternative drugs should be considered first.

disinfectants easily inactivate the organism. Laboratory workers should not attempt to grow the organism unless working under BSL-3 conditions.

PROPHYLAXIS

Vaccine. An investigational (IND) live-attenuated vaccine (live vaccine strain – LVS), administered by scarification, has been given to > 5,000 persons without significant adverse reactions. It prevents typhoidal, and ameliorates ulceroglandular, forms of laboratory-acquired tularemia. Aerosol challenge tests in animals and human volunteers have demonstrated significant protection. As with all vaccines, the degree of protection depends upon the magnitude of the challenge dose. Vaccine-induced protection could be overwhelmed by extremely high doses of the tularemia bacterium. Currently, no effective licensed vaccine is available in developed nations.

- **Immunoprophylaxis.** There is no passive immunoprophylaxis (i.e., immune globulin) available for pre- or postexposure management of tularemia.
- **Preexposure chemoprophylaxis.** No antibiotics are licensed by the FDA for use before exposure to tularemia. However, chemoprophylaxis with ciprofloxacin or doxycycline may protect against tularemia based upon in vitro susceptibilities.

Postexposure chemoprophylaxis.

Preferred

- **Doxycycline** 100 mg PO bid for adults and children 45 kg (for children < 45kg use 2.2 mg / kg PO bid), or
- **Ciprofloxacin** 500 mg PO bid for adults (15 mg/kg PO bid (up to 1 gm/d) for children)

Postexposure chemoprophylaxis should ideally begin with 24 h of exposure and continue for at least 14 d. These oral antibiotic dosages may also be appropriate for treatment in mass casualty settings in which IV antibiotics are not available.

Chemoprophylaxis is generally not recommended after potential natural (tick bite, rabbit, or other animal) exposures.

VIRAL AGENTS

Viruses are considered the simplest microorganisms, consisting of genetic material, either RNA or DNA, surrounded by a protein coat. In some cases, the viral particle is also surrounded by an outer lipid bilayer. Viruses are much smaller than bacteria and vary in size from 0.02 µmm to 0.2 µmm (1 µmm = 1/1000 mm). Viruses are intracellular parasites and lack a system for their own metabolism. Therefore, they require host cell synthetic machinery for replication and survival, which means that unlike bacteria, viruses, cannot be cultivated in synthetic nutritive solutions. The types of host cells that viruses infect include animal, plant, and even bacteria. Because a very specific interaction occurs between the virus and the host cell, every virus requires its own special type of host cell for replication. Virus replication usually brings about changes in the host cell that eventually lead to cell death. To produce a large amount of virus, either host cells cultivated in synthetic nutrient solutions or chorioallantoic membranes of fertilized eggs can be used. Ultimately, the synthetic production of viruses requires a large amount of resources to include time and money. This handbook covers three types of viruses which could potentially be employed as bioagents: smallpox, alphaviruses (e.g., VEE), and hemorrhagic fever viruses.

Smallpox (Variola)

SUMMARY

Signs and Symptoms: Acute clinical manifestations begin with malaise, fever, rigors, vomiting, headache, and backache. Two to 3 days later, skin lesions appear, quickly progress from macules to papules, and eventually to pustular vesicles. They are "centrifugal" (more abundant on the extremities and face), and the stages develop synchronously.

Diagnosis: Initially, must be clinical. Neither electron nor light microscopy is capable of discriminating *Variola* (smallpox) from vaccinia, monkeypox, or cowpox. Polymerase chain reaction (PCR) diagnostic techniques are more accurate in discriminating *Variola* and other orthopoxviruses.

Treatment: At present, there is no FDA-approved chemotherapy, but three IND products have demonstrated efficacy in *Orthopox* animal models including *Variola*, and have been used to treat disseminated vaccinia infection under an emergency IND (EIND), and treatment of a clinical case remains mainly supportive.

Prophylaxis: Immediate vaccination or revaccination should be instituted for all personnel exposed. This is most effective during the first 4 days after exposure.

Isolation and Decontamination: Patients should be considered infectious from onset of rash until all scabs separate and should be isolated using both droplet and airborne precautions during this period. In the civilian setting, strict quarantine of asymptomatic contacts for 17 days after exposure may prove to be impractical to enforce. A reasonable alternative would be to require contacts to check their temperatures daily. Any fever above 38°C (101°F) during the 17 days after exposure to a confirmed case would suggest the development of smallpox. The contact should then be isolated immediately, ideally at home, until the diagnosis is either confirmed or ruled out and remain in isolation until all scabs separate.

OVERVIEW

Smallpox was caused by an *Orthopoxvirus*, *Variola*, which is known to exist in at least two strains, *Variola major* (10 to 30% mortality) and the milder *Variola minor* (< 1% mortality). Despite the global eradication of smallpox and continued availability of a vaccine, the potential weaponization of *Variola* may continue to pose a military threat. This threat may be attributed to the aerosol infectivity of the virus, the relative ease of large-scale production, and an increasingly *Orthopoxvirus*-naive populace. Although the fully developed cutaneous eruption of smallpox is unique, earlier stages of the rash could be mistaken for chicken pox (varicella). Secondary spread of infection constitutes a nosocomial hazard from the time of onset of a patient's exanthem until scabs have separated. Quarantine should be applied to secondary contacts for 17 days postexposure. Vaccination and vaccinia immune globulin each possess some efficacy in postexposure prophylaxis. Three antivirals (cidofovir, ST-246 and CMX001), currently IND products, may also be of benefit but are not currently licensed and would have to be used under an EIND.

HISTORY AND SIGNIFICANCE

Endemic smallpox was declared eradicated in 1980 by the World Health Organization (WHO). Although two WHO-approved repositories of *Variola* virus remain at the Centers for Disease Control and Prevention (CDC) in Atlanta and at the Russian State Centre for Research on Virology and Biotechnology (Koltsovo, Novosibirsk Region) Russian Federation, the extent of clandestine stockpiles in other parts of the world remains unknown. The WHO Advisory Committee on *Variola* virus research recommended that all stocks of smallpox be destroyed by 30 June 2002. However, destruction has been delayed annually since that time by the WHO Health Assembly due to concerns over the need for further study of the virus given its potential as a biological warfare agent.

The U.S. ended routine smallpox military vaccination in 1989, but began vaccination again in 2003 for troops deployed to Southwest Asia and the Republic of Korea. Routine civilian vaccination in the United States was discontinued in 1972. Thus much of the population is now susceptible to *Variola major. Variola* may have been used by the British Army against Native Americans and later against the rebelling American colonials during the eighteenth century. Japan considered the use of smallpox as a biowarfare in World War II and it has been considered as a possible threat agent against U.S. forces for many years. In addition, the former Soviet Union is reported to have produced and stockpiled massive quantities of the virus for use as a biological weapon. It is unknown whether any of these stockpiles may still exist in Russia or elsewhere.

The full-length sequence of several *Variola* strains have been published. Rapid advances in synthetic biology now make it at least theoretically possible to construct it solely from fragments produced utilizing a DNA synthesizer The construction of a *Mycoplasma* that is three times larger than *Variola* has demonstrated the feasibility of such an accomplishment. Thus the old strategy of closely supervising existing stocks of *Variola* no longer ensures that a determined adversary could not obtain *Variola*.

CLINICAL FEATURES

The incubation period of naturally acquired smallpox averages 12 days, although it could range from 7-19 days after exposure. Clinical manifestations begin with malaise, high fever (to 104°F), rigors, vomiting, headache, backache, and prostration; 15% of patients develop delirium. Approximately 10% of light-skinned patients exhibit an erythematous rash during this phase. Two to 3 days later, an enanthem consisting of small, painful ulcerations of the tongue and oropharynx appears simultaneously with (or within 24 h of) a discrete rash about the face, hands, and forearms.

After development of eruptions on the lower extremities, the rash spreads centrally to the trunk over the next week. The exanthem typically begins as small, erythematous macules which progress to 2-3-mm papules over 2 to 3 days, then to 2-5-mm vesicles within 1 to 2 more days. Four to 7 days after rash onset, the vesicles become 4-6 mm umbilicated pustules, often accompanied by a second, smaller fever spike. Lesions are more abundant on the extremities and face, and this "centrifugal" distribution is an important diagnostic feature. In distinct contrast to varicella, lesions on various segments of the body remain generally synchronous in their stages of development. From 8 to 14 dats after onset, the pustules form scabs that leave depressed depigmented scars upon healing. Death, if it occurs, is usually during the second week of clinical disease. The precise cause of death is not entirely understood, but was historically attributed to toxemia, with high levels of circulating immune complexes. Although *Variola* concentrations in the throat, conjunctiva, and urine diminish with time, the virus can be readily recovered from scabs throughout convalescence. Therefore, patients should be isolated and considered infectious until all scabs separate.

In the 20th century, two distinct types of smallpox were recognized. *Variola minor* was distinguished by milder systemic toxicity and more diminutive pox lesions, and caused a 1% case fatality rate (CFR) in unvaccinated victims. However, the prototypical disease caused by *Variola major* resulted in a CFR of 3% and 30% in the vaccinated and unvaccinated, respectively. CFRs were higher in certain populations (e.g., Pacific islanders and Native Americans), at extremes of age, during pregnancy (average 65% for ordinary smallpox), and in people with immunodeficiencies. Greater mortality was associated with higher concentrations of lesions, with confluence of lesions portending the worst prognosis. Smallpox during pregnancy resulted in an increased incidence of spontaneous abortions. Acute complications of smallpox included viral keratitis or secondary ocular infection (1%), encephalitis (<1%), and arthritis (up to 2% of children). Bronchopneumonia was also in severely ill patients.

Other clinical forms of *Variola major* - flat-type and hemorrhagic-type smallpox - were notable for severe mortality. Flat-type smallpox occurred in about 6% of all cases and was most common in children. Hemorrhagic smallpox occurred in about 2-3% of all cases, was more common in pregnant women and the immunocompromised, and presented with both "early" and "late" forms. Early hemorrhagic disease had a shorter incubation period, often large areas of ecchymosis, and fulminant progression to death, sometimes before lesions had even formed. In the late form, the disease progression was normal, with discrete hemorrhagic areas forming at lesion sites. CFRs were approximately 95% in both flat and hemorrhagic forms.

Partially immune patients, especially those vaccinated several years before smallpox exposure, could develop less severe forms of disease. This modified smallpox is a clinical form of disease characterized by fewer lesions which are more superficial, associated with a less pronounced fever and a more rapid resolution of disease, often with lesion crusting within 10 days of onset. Some previously immune individuals or infants with maternal antibodies could develop a short-lived febrile syndrome without rash upon exposure to smallpox.

Long-term sequelae in survivors of smallpox include blindness from corneal scarring (1-4%), growth abnormalities in children, and disfiguring or even physically debilitating dermal scarring.

Animal studies suggest that unnaturally large inhaled inoculae of poxvirus may result in a significantly shortened incubation period (even as little as 3-5 d) and fulminant pulmonary disease with or without appearance of rash before death; the implications of these findings for human disease resulting from intentional smallpox aerosolization are unknown at this time.

Historically, smallpox tended to spread slowly through communities. Smallpox could become endemic in densely populated regions even in a population with up to 80% vaccination rates. Increased person to person spread of disease was associated with: 1) exposure to cases with confluent rash or severe enanthem; 2) exposure to cases with severe bronchiolitis and cough; 3) low humidity environment; 4) crowding (as in winter or rainy seasons). The average secondary attack rate of *Variola major* was 58.4% in unvaccinated household contacts and 3.8% in vaccinated household contacts.

A relative of *Variola*, monkeypox, occurs naturally in equatorial Africa. In 2003, an outbreak of 81 primary human cases occurred in the U.S. due to exposure to exotic pets, some of which had been imported from Africa. Descriptions of human monkeypox in Africa reveal a disease that could be clinically indistinguishable from smallpox with the exception of a generally lower CFR and notable cervical and inguinal lymphadenopathy appearing 1-2 d before the rash in 90% of cases. The U.S. cases in 2003 tended to be less severe, with often localized lesions only, no deaths, and no secondary transmission to other humans.

DIAGNOSIS

Smallpox must be distinguished from other vesicular exanthems, such as chickenpox, erythema multiforme with bullae, and allergic contact dermatitis. In a confirmed outbreak, smallpox would likely be a clinical diagnosis. Particularly problematic to the necessary infection control measures would be the failure to recognize relatively mild cases of smallpox in persons with partial immunity, or extremely severe cases in patients without classical disease. Therefore, isolation of suspected cases, quarantine of potential exposures, and initiation of medical countermeasures should be promptly followed by an accurate laboratory diagnosis. Providers who collect or process specimens should be vaccinated and should implement contact and airborne precautions. Specimens should be collected only upon the direction of public health officials, who will provide further guidance. Typical *Variola* specimens might include scrapings of skin lesions, lesion fluid, crusts, blood, or pharyngeal swabs. CDC has prepared a poster and diagnostic algorithm (http://www.bt.cdc.gov/agent/smallpox/diagnosis/pdf/spox-poster-full.pdf) to assist in decision making.

A method of presumptive diagnosis is the demonstration of characteristic poxvirus virions on electron microscopy of vesicular scrapings. Under light microscopy, aggregations of *Variola* virus particles, called Guarnieri bodies, can be seen. Another rapid but relatively insensitive test for Guarnieri bodies in vesicular scrapings is Gispen's modified silver stain, in which cytoplasmic inclusions appear black. However, none of the above laboratory tests is capable of discriminating *Variola* from vaccinia, monkeypox, or cowpox.

Diagnosis of *Variola* has classically required isolation of the virus and characterization of its growth on chicken egg chorioallantoic membranes. Real-time PCR assays are now available and provide a rapid and specific diagnosis. Specific smallpox PCR diagnosis is presently available only at Laboratory Response Network (LRN) national laboratories (CDC and USAMRIID) under BSL-4 conditions. A real-time PCR assay that detects all orthopoxviruses (including vaccinia) may be available from the Army Medical Laboratory (AML) for a presumptive diagnosis.

Neutralizing antibodies to *Variola* form in the first week of illness and may persist for many years. Hemaglutination-inhibition antibodies are detectible by the 16th day of infection and complement fixation antibodies by the 18th, but both begin to decrease after 1 yr.

Associated laboratory findings, including the complete blood counts (CBC) of patients with ordinary smallpox, often exhibited a neutropenia and lymphocytosis during the eruptive stage. Neutrophils could become elevated during the late pustular stage when secondary bacterial infections would occur. Mild thrombocytopenia was common. In hemorrhagic smallpox, thrombocytopenia was progressive and severe as disseminated intravascular coagulation developed.

MEDICAL MANAGEMENT

Medical personnel must be able to recognize a vesicular exanthem and consider the etiology as potentially *Variola*, and then quickly initiate appropriate countermeasures. Any confirmed case of human smallpox should be considered an international emergency with immediate reporting to public health authorities. People who have been exposed to known cases of smallpox should be monitored for a minimum of 17 days from exposure regardless of their vaccination status; such individuals should be immediately isolated using droplet and airborne precautions at the onset of fever. In a civilian setting, strict quarantine of asymptomatic contacts may prove to be impractical to enforce. A reasonable alternative would be to require contacts to remain at home and to check their temperatures daily. Any fever above 38°C (101°F) during the 17 days after exposure to a confirmed case would suggest the development of smallpox. The contact should then be isolated immediately, preferably at home, until smallpox is either confirmed or ruled out and remain in isolation until all scabs separate. Patients should be considered infectious until all scabs separate. Immediate vaccination or revaccination should also be undertaken for all personnel exposed to either weaponized *Variola* virus or a clinical case of smallpox. Caregivers should be vaccinated and continue to wear appropriate personal protective equipment regardless of vaccination status. Weaponized smallpox strains encountered in the future may be genetically altered to render the current vaccine ineffective, a possibility experimentally validated in similar poxvirus animal models.

The potential for airborne spread to other than close contacts is controversial. In general, close person-to-person contact is required for transmission to reliably occur. Nevertheless, *Variola*'s potential for airborne spread in conditions of low relative humidity was demonstrated during two hospital outbreaks. Indirect transmission by contaminated bedding or by other fomites was infrequent. Some close contacts harbored virus in their throats without developing disease and hence might have served as a means of secondary transmission.

Vaccination with a verified clinical "take" (vesicle with subsequent scar formation) within the past 3 yrs is considered to render a person immune to smallpox. However, given the difficulties and uncertainties under wartime conditions of verifying the adequacy of troops' prior vaccination, routine revaccination of all potentially exposed personnel would seem prudent if there existed a significant prospect of smallpox exposure.

Antivirals for use against smallpox are under investigation. Cidofovir has had significant *in vitro* and *in vivo* activity in animal studies. Whether it would offer benefit superior to immediate postexposure vaccination in humans has not been determined. While cidofovir is a licensed drug for intravenous administration, its use for treating smallpox is "off-label" and it should be administered as an IND (See Appendix L for guidelines on the administration of INDs). Topical antivirals such as trifluridine or idoxuridine may be useful for treating smallpox ocular disease but are difficult to obtain. Two new oral antivirals ST-246 and CMX001 (prodrug of cidofovir), are under investigation and have been utilized under "compassionate use" (i.e., "single use") IND requests to treat a limited number of severe cases of vaccinia. Data from non-human primate models of *Variola* and monkeypox have shown efficacy of ST-246 and cidofovir.

Supportive care is imperative for successful management of smallpox patients; measures include maintenance of hydration and nutrition, pain control, and management of secondary infections.

PROPHYLAXIS

Vaccine: Smallpox vaccine (made from vaccinia virus) is most often administered by intradermal inoculation with a bifurcated needle, a process that became known as "scarification" because of the permanent scar that resulted. The current smallpox vaccine is *ACAM2000*, which is a licensed product, and unlike previous smallpox vaccines, is produced in cell culture. Primary vaccinees receive three punctures with the needle, repeat vaccinees receive 15. Vaccination after exposure to smallpox may prevent or ameliorate disease if given as soon as possible and preferably within 4 d after exposure. A vesicle typically appears at the vaccination site 5-7 days after inoculation, with associated erythema and induration. The lesion forms a scab and gradually heals over the next 1-2 weeks; the evolution of the lesion may be more rapid, with less severe symptoms, in those with previous immunity.

Smallpox vaccination side effects include low-grade fever and axillary lymphadenopathy. The attendant erythema and induration of the vaccination vesicle is frequently misdiagnosed as bacterial superinfection. More severe vaccine reactions (more common in primary vaccinees) include inadvertent inoculation of the virus to other sites such as the face, eyelid, or other persons (~ 6/10,000 vaccinees), and generalized vaccinia, which is a systemic spread of the virus to produce mucocutaneous lesions away from the primary vaccination site (~3/10,000 vaccinees). Approximately 1/10,000 primary vaccinees will experience a transient, acute myopericarditis. Rare, but often fatal, adverse reactions include *eczema vaccinatum* (generalized cutaneous spread of vaccinia in patients with eczema), progressive vaccinia (systemic spread of vaccinia in immunocompromised individuals), and post-vaccinia encephalitis.

Vaccination is *contraindicated* in the following conditions unless a smallpox outbreak is documented: immunosuppression, HIV infection, history or evidence of eczema, other active severe skin disorders, pregnancy, or current household, sexual, or other close physical contact with person(s) possessing one of these conditions. In addition, vaccination should not be performed in breastfeeding mothers, in individuals with serious cardiovascular disease or with three risk factors for cardiovascular disease, or individuals who are using topical steroid eye medications or who have had recent eye surgery. Despite these caveats, most authorities, including current CDC guidelines, state that, with the exception of significant impairment of systemic immunity, there are no absolute contraindications to postexposure vaccination of a person who experiences *bona fide* exposure to *Variola*. However, concomitant vaccine immune globulin administration is recommended for pregnant and eczematous persons in such circumstances.

Passive Immunoprophylaxis: Vaccinia immune globulin (VIG) is indicated for some complications to the smallpox (vaccinia) vaccine (generalized vaccinia with systemic illness, ocular vaccinia without keratitis, *eczema vaccinatum*, and progressive vaccinia), and should be available when administering vaccine. It is available as an IND through both DoD and the CDC in IM and IV formulations. A formulation of VIG-IV has been licensed, but is currently in very limited supply. The dose for prophylaxis or treatment is 100 mg/kg for the IV formulation (first line). If VIG-intravenous is not available, cidofovir may be of use for treating vaccinia adverse events (second line). The intramuscular VIG formulation (VIG-IM) is dosed 0.6 ml/kg (third line). Due to the large volume of the IM formulation (42 ml in a 70 kg person), the dose would be given in multiple sites over 24-36 h. Limited data suggest that VIG may also be of value in post-exposure prophylaxis of smallpox when given within the first week after exposure, and concurrently with vaccination. Vaccination alone is recommended for those without contraindications to the vaccine. If greater than 1 week has elapsed after exposure, administration of both products (vaccine and VIG), if available, is reasonable.

Venezuelan Equine Encephalitis (VEE)

SUMMARY

Signs and Symptoms: Incubation period is 2-6 days. VEE presents as an acute systemic febrile illness in which encephalitis develops in a small percentage (4% children; < 1% adults). Symptoms include generalized malaise, spiking fevers, rigors, severe headache, photophobia, and myalgias for 24-72 h. Nausea, vomiting, cough, sore throat, and diarrhea may follow. Full recovery from malaise and fatigue takes 1-2 weeks. The incidence of CNS disease and associated morbidity and mortality could be much higher after a biowarfare attack with VEE.

Diagnosis: Clinical and epidemiological diagnosis. Physical findings are nonspecific. The white blood cell count may show a leukopenia with striking lymphopenia. Virus may be isolated from serum, and in some cases throat or nasal swab specimens. Both neutralizing and IgG antibody in paired sera or VEE-specific IgM present in a single serum sample indicates recent infection.

Treatment: Supportive only. Treat uncomplicated VEE infections with analgesics to relieve headache and myalgia. Patients who develop encephalitis may require anticonvulsants and intensive supportive care to maintain fluid and electrolyte balance, ensure adequate ventilation, and avoid complicating secondary bacterial infections.

Prophylaxis: A live, attenuated vaccine is available as an IND. A second, formalin-inactivated, killed vaccine is available for boosting antibody titers in those initially receiving the first vaccine. There is no postexposure immunoprophylaxis. In experimental animals, alpha-interferon and the interferon-inducer poly-ICLC have proven highly effective as postexposure prophylaxis.

Isolation and Decontamination: Patient isolation and quarantine are not required. Standard precautions augmented with vector control while the patient is febrile. There is no evidence of direct human-to-human or horse-to-human transmission. The virus can be destroyed by heat (80°C for 30 min) and standard disinfectants.

OVERVIEW

The Venezuelan equine encephalitis (VEE) virus complex is a group of six serotypes (I to VI) which contain 13 serologically distinct subtypes that are endemic in northern South America and Trinidad and cause rare cases of human encephalitis in Central America, Mexico, and Florida. These viruses can cause severe diseases in humans and equids (horses, mules, burros, and donkeys). Natural infections are acquired by the bites of a wide variety of mosquitoes. Equids serve as amplifying hosts and sources of mosquito infection.

Western and eastern equine encephalitis (WEE and EEE) viruses are similar to the VEE virus complex, are often difficult to distinguish clinically, and share similar aspects of transmission and epidemiology. The human infective dose for VEE virus is thought to be approximately 10-100 organisms, which is one of the principal reasons that the VEE virus is considered a potentially effective bioagent. Neither the population density of infected mosquitoes nor the aerosol concentration of viral particles has to be great to allow significant transmission of VEE virus in a biowarfare attack. There is no evidence of direct human-to-human or horse-to-human transmission. Natural aerosol transmission is not known to occur. VEE particles are not considered stable in the environment, and are thus not as persistent as the bacteria responsible for Q fever, tularemia, or anthrax. Heat and standard disinfectants can easily kill VEE viruses.

HISTORY AND SIGNIFICANCE

Initially isolated from moribund horses in 1938, VEE virus was shown to be capable of causing disease in humans as well in 1952 by researchers in Colombia. Between 1969 and 1971, an epizootic of a "highly pathogenic strain" of VEE virus emerged in Guatemala, moved through Mexico, and entered Texas in June 1971. This strain was virulent in both equids and humans. In Mexico, there were 8,000-10,000 equine deaths, "tens of thousands" of equine cases, and 17,000 human cases (but no human deaths). Over 10,000 horses in Texas died. Once the Texas border was breached, a national emergency was declared and resources were mobilized to vaccinate horses in 20 states. Ninety-five percent of all horses and donkeys were vaccinated; over 3.2 million animals. In addition equine quarantines were established and control of mosquito populations was obtained with the use of broad-scale insecticides along the Rio Grande Valley and the Gulf Coast. After this outbreak there was an almost 20-yr break with no confirmed VEE activity. Several small outbreaks were recorded beginning in 1992 in localized areas. A large VEE outbreak occurred in 1995 in Venezuela and Columbia involving over 75,000 human cases and as many as 300 deaths.

VEE is better characterized than EEE or WEE, primarily because it was tested as a biowarfare agent during the U.S. offensive biowarfare program in the 1950s and 1960s. Other countries have, or are suspected to have, weaponized this agent. In compliance with President Richard Nixon's National Security Decision Memorandum 35 of November 1969 directing the destruction of the existing stocks of U.S. biological and chemical weapons, all VEE virus weapon stocks were destroyed under supervision.

These viruses could theoretically be produced in large amounts in either a wet or dried form by relatively unsophisticated and inexpensive systems. This form of VEE virus could be intentionally disseminated as an aerosol and would be highly infectious. It could also be spread by the purposeful dissemination of infected mosquitoes, which likely transmit the virus throughout their lives (the dark rice field mosquito, *Psorophora columbiae*, is the only mosquito confirmed to transmit VEE from horse-to-mosquito-to-horse in the Texas epidemic cycle). The VEE complex viruses are relatively stable during the storage and manipulation procedures necessary for weaponization.

Natural human epidemics are almost always preceded by epizootics, characterized by severe and often fatal (30-90%) encephalitic outbreaks in equids. However, a biowarfare attack with virus intentionally disseminated as an aerosol would most likely cause human disease as a primary event or simultaneously with equids. Occasionally during natural epidemics, illness or death in wild or free-ranging equids may not be recognized before the onset of human disease, therefore a natural epidemic could be confused with a biowarfare event, and data on the onset of disease should be considered with caution. A more reliable method for determining the likelihood of an intentional event would be the presence of VEE outside of its natural geographic range. A biowarfare attack in a region populated by equids and appropriate mosquito vectors could initiate an epizootic / epidemic.

CLINICAL FEATURES

Susceptibility in humans is high (90-100%), and nearly 100% of those infected develop overt illness. The overall case fatality rate for VEE is less than 1%, although it is somewhat higher in the very young or aged. Recovery from an infection results in excellent short-term and long-term immunity to the infective strain, but may not protect against other strains of the virus.

VEE is primarily an acute, incapacitating, febrile illness with encephalitis developing in only a small percentage of the infected population. Most VEE infections are mild (in contrast to clinically apparent EEE and WEE infection, in which encephalitis is common). After an incubation period as short as 28 h but typically 2-6 days, onset of prostrating illness is usually sudden. This acute phase of illness is often manifested by generalized malaise, chills, spiking high fevers (38°C-40.5°C), rigors, severe headache, photophobia, and myalgias prominent in the legs and lumbosacral area. Nausea, vomiting, and diarrhea are also common. Physical signs may include tachycardia, conjunctival injection, erythematous pharynx, and muscle tenderness. Severe symptoms generally subside within 2-4 days, to be followed by asthenia (malaise and fatigue) lasting for 1-2 wks before full recovery. A biphasic illness, with recurrence of the acute symptoms 4-8 d after initial onset of disease, has been described infrequently. If severe encephalitis develops, clinical signs may include neck rigidity, altered states of consciousness, and convulsions. Generally, about 10% of patients in natural epidemics will be ill enough to require hospitalization.

During natural epidemics, approximately 4% of infected children (<15 yrs old) and less than 1% of adults will develop signs of severe CNS infection. In those that develop severe neurological illness, case fatality rates (CFRs) have been reported as high as 35% in children and 10% in adults. Adults rarely develop neurologic complications during natural infections. Mild CNS findings would include lethargy, somnolence, photophobia or mild confusion, with or without nuchal rigidity. Seizures, ataxia, paralysis, or coma follow more severe CNS involvement. Experimental aerosol challenges in animals suggest that the incidence of CNS disease and associated morbidity and mortality could be much higher after a biowarfare attack, as the VEE virus may travel along the olfactory nerve and spread directly to the CNS and result in acute neurological signs. School-age children may be more susceptible to a fulminant form of the disease characterized by depletion of lymphoid tissues, encephalitis, interstitial pneumonitis, and hepatitis, which follows a lethal course over 48-72 h. VEE during pregnancy may cause encephalitis in the fetus, placental damage, spontaneous abortion, or severe congenital neuroanatomical anomalies.

DIAGNOSIS

A diagnosis of VEE is suspected on clinical and epidemiological grounds, but confirmed by virus isolation, serology, electrochemiluminescence (ECL), or PCR. A variety of serological tests are applicable, including IgM, ELISA, indirect fluorescent antibody, hemagglutination inhibition, complement-fixation, and IgG. For persons without prior known exposure to VEE complex viruses, a presumptive diagnosis may be made by identifying IgM antibody in a single serum sample taken 5-7 days after onset of illness. PCR procedures are available for confirmation, but are generally available only as a rear echelon laboratory capability.

Samples suitable for performing diagnostic tests include blood culture (only in appropriate BSL-3 containment), acute and convalescent sera, and cerebrospinal fluid. Viremia during the acute phase of the illness (but not during encephalitis) is generally high enough to allow detection by antigen-capture ELISA or ECL. Virus isolation is time consuming, but may be performed from serum and throat or nasal swab specimens collected in the first 3 days of illness by inoculation of cell cultures or suckling mice (a gold standard identification assay for VEE virus). VEE virus should be isolated only in a BSL-3 laboratory.

The white blood cell count is often normal at the onset of symptoms and then usually shows a leukopenia with a striking lymphopenia, and sometimes a mild thrombocytopenia by the second to third day of illness. Each of these abnormalities will usually resolve over the ensuing 1-2 weeks. Temporary, mild elevations of lactate dehydrogenase (LDH), aspartate transaminase (AST), and alkaline phosphatase (ALP) may also be present. In patients with encephalitis, the CSF pressure may be increased and contain up to 1,000 white blood cells / mm^3 (predominantly mononuclear cells) and a mildly elevated protein concentration.

An outbreak of VEE may be difficult to distinguish from influenza on clinical grounds. Clues to the diagnosis might include the appearance of a small proportion of neurological cases, lack of person-to-person spread, or disease in equines. A biowarfare aerosol attack could lead to an epidemic of febrile meningoencephalitis featuring seizures and coma. In a biowarfare context, the differential diagnosis would include other causes of aseptic meningitis and meningoencephalitis.

MEDICAL MANAGEMENT

No specific antiviral therapy exists; hence treatment is supportive only. Patients with uncomplicated VEE may be treated with analgesics to relieve headache and myalgia. Nausea and emesis can lead to dehydration and necessitate IV fluids in some cases. Patients who develop encephalitis may require anticonvulsants and intensive supportive care to maintain fluid and electrolyte balance, ensure adequate ventilation, and avoid complicating secondary bacterial infections. In the presence of mosquito vectors, patients should be treated in a screened room or in quarters treated with a residual insecticide for at least 5 days after onset, or until afebrile, as human cases may be infectious for mosquitoes for at least 72 h. Patient isolation and quarantine are otherwise not required; sufficient contagion control is provided by implementing standard precautions augmented with vector control while the patient is febrile. Patient-to-patient transmission by means of respiratory droplet infection has not been shown to occur. The virus can be destroyed by heat (80°C for 30 min) and standard disinfectants.

PROPHYLAXIS

Vaccine: There are two unlicensed (IND) VEE vaccines that have been administered to humans. The first investigational vaccine (designated TC-83) was developed in the 1960s and is a live, attenuated cell-culture-propagated vaccine produced by the Salk Institute. This vaccine is not effective against all of the serotypes in the VEE complex. It has been used to protect several thousand persons against laboratory infections and is presently licensed for use in equids (and was used in the 1970-71 Texas epizootic in horses), but is an IND vaccine for humans. It is given as a single 0.5-ml subcutaneous dose. Fever, malaise, and headache occur in approximately 20% of vaccinees, and may be moderate to severe in 10% of those necessitating bed rest for 1-2 days. Another 18% of vaccinees fail to develop detectable neutralizing antibodies, but it is unknown whether they are susceptible to later infection. Contraindications for use include a concurrent viral infection or pregnancy. Individuals with diabetes or a close family history of diabetes should not receive this vaccine.

A second IND vaccine (designated C-84) has also been tested, but not licensed, in humans and is prepared by formalin-inactivation of the TC-83 strain. This vaccine is not used for primary vaccination, but is used to boost non-responders to TC-83. Administer 0.5 ml subcutaneously at 2-4 week intervals for up to three inoculations or until an antibody response is measured. Periodic boosters are required. The C-84 vaccine alone does not protect rodents against experimental aerosol challenge. Therefore, C-84 is used only as a booster immunogen for the TC-83 vaccine.

As with all vaccines, the degree of protection depends upon the magnitude of the challenge dose; vaccine-induced protection could be overwhelmed by extremely high inocula of the pathogen. Research is underway to produce an improved, second-generation VEE vaccine.

Immunoprophylaxis: At present, there is no licensed preexposure or postexposure immunoprophylatic. In animal models, protection from subcutaneous and aerosolized VEE virus has been demonstrated by passive transfer of neutralizing monoclonal antibodies administered 24 h pre- or 24 h postinfection.

Chemoprophylaxis: In experimental animals, alpha-interferon and the interferon-inducer poly-ICLC have proven highly effective for postexposure chemoprophylaxis of VEE. There are no clinical data on which to assess efficacy of these drugs in humans.

Viral Hemorrhagic Fevers (VHFs)

SUMMARY

Signs and Symptoms: Viral hemorrhagic fevers (VHFs) are illnesses characterized by fever and bleeding diathesis. Manifestations of VHF often include flushing of the face and chest, petechiae, frank bleeding, edema, hypotension, and shock. Malaise, myalgias, headache, vomiting, and diarrhea occur frequently.

Diagnosis: Definitive diagnosis is usually made at a reference laboratory with advanced biocontainment capability. An early clinical diagnosis is crucial for appropriate management and to minimize potential nosocomial spread. Any patient with a compatible clinical syndrome should suggest the possibility of a VHF.

Treatment: Intensive supportive care may be required. Antiviral therapy with IV ribavirin may be useful in *Bunyaviridae* and *Arenaviridae* infections (specifically Lassa fever, Crimean-Congo hemorrhagic fever, and hemorrhagic fever with renal syndrome due to Old World hantavirus infection) and should be used only under an Investigational New Drug (IND) protocol. Convalescent plasma may be effective in Argentine or Bolivian hemorrhagic fevers (available only as INDs).

Prophylaxis: The only licensed VHF vaccine is the 17D yellow fever vaccine. Experimental vaccines for other VHFs are not readily available. Prophylactic ribavirin may be effective for some *Bunyaviridae* and *Arenaviridae* infections (available only as an IND).

Isolation and Decontamination: All VHF patients should be cared for under strict contact precautions, including hand hygiene double gloves, gowns, shoe and leg coverings, and face shield or goggles. Airborne precautions should be instituted to the maximum extent possible and especially for procedures that induce aerosols (e.g., bronchoscopy). At a minimum, a fit-tested, HEPA filter-equipped respirator (such as an N-95 mask), a battery-powered, air-purifying respirator (PAPR), or a positive pressure-supplied air respirator should be worn by personnel sharing an enclosed space with or coming within 6 feet of a VHF patient. Multiple patients should stay in a separate building or a ward with an isolated air-handling system when feasible. Ideally, VHF patients should be isolated in a negative-pressure isolation room with 6-12 air exchanges per h. Environmental decontamination is accomplished with hypochlorite or phenolic disinfectants.

OVERVIEW

The VHFs are a diverse group of illnesses caused by lipid-enveloped, single-stranded RNA viruses from four viral families: *Arenaviridae, Bunyaviridae, Filoviridae,* and *Flaviviridae.* They are unified by their potential to present as a severe febrile illness accompanied by shock and a hemorrhagic diathesis. The *Arenaviridae* include the etiologic agents of Lassa fever and Argentine (Junin), Bolivian (Machupo), and Venezuelan (Sabia) hemorrhagic fevers. The *Bunyaviridae* include the members of the *Hantavirus* genus that cause hemorrhagic fever with renal syndrome (HFRS); the Congo-Crimean hemorrhagic fever virus from the *Nairovirus* genus; and the Rift Valley fever virus from the *Phlebovirus* genus. The *Filoviridae* include Ebola and Marburg viruses. Finally, the *Flaviviridae* include dengue, yellow fever, and two viruses in the tick-borne encephalitis group that cause VHF, Omsk hemorrhagic fever virus and Kyasanur Forest disease virus. These viruses are spread in a variety of ways, frequently through blood/body fluid exposure, and most have zoonotic potential (transmission from animals to humans by a vector, inhalation or ingestion of excretions/secretions of rodents); some may be transmitted to humans through a respiratory portal of entry. Although historic evidence for weaponization does not exist for many of these viruses, they are included in this handbook because of their *potential* for aerosol dissemination, weaponization, or likelihood for confusion with similar agents that might be weaponized.

HISTORY AND SIGNIFICANCE

Because these viruses are so diverse and occur in different endemic geographic locations, a comprehensive discussion is beyond the scope of this handbook. However, each viral infection possesses a number of different features that may provide insight into their possible importance as biological threat agents.

Arenaviridae: Lassa virus causes Lassa fever in West Africa, where endemic transmission is related to infected natal multimammate mice (*Mastomys natalensis*), a common rodent in equatorial Africa. Over 5,000 deaths in West Africa are attributed to Lassa each year, with between 200,000 – 300,000 annual infections. Argentine hemorrhagic fever (AHF) is caused by Junin virus and was first described in 1955 among field workers who harvested corn. Typically, 300 to 600 cases per year occur in areas of the Argentine pampas. Bolivian, Brazilian, and Venezuelan hemorrhagic fevers are caused by the related Machupo, Guanarito, and Sabia viruses, respectively. Arena viruses are transmitted from their rodent reservoirs to humans through inhalation of dusts contaminated with rodent excreta. Nosocomial transmission is probably possible with all *Arenavirus* infections but is frequently a problem with Lassa fever. Lassa infection of healthcare workers has been attributed to parenteral exposures, contact with body fluids, and aerosols generated by patients.

Bunyaviridae: Congo-Crimean hemorrhagic fever (CCHF) is a tick-borne disease with a widespread distribution from sub-Saharan Africa through southeastern Europe, Central Asia and the Indian sub-continent. It may also be spread by contact with the body fluids or slaughtered meat of infected animals and in health-care settings. The 2009 death of a U.S. soldier who was infected with CCHF while stationed in Afghanistan was a reminder of the ongoing endemic disease risk in certain parts of the world. Rift Valley fever (RVF) is a mosquito-borne disease that occurs in Central and East Africa but can also be transmitted by handling infected tissues (animal slaughter), ingestion of raw milk, and by aerosol (particularly laboratory workers). In 2000, a large outbreak occurred outside Africa in Yemen and Saudi Arabia. RVF is not only on the U.S. Department of Health and Human Services select agent list like most VHFs but it is also listed on the U.S. Department of Agriculture select agent list as an agent that deleteriously affects animals of agricultural significance. The hantaviruses are rodent-borne viruses with a wide geographic distribution. Hantaan and closely related Old World hantaviruses cause hemorrhagic fever with renal syndrome (HFRS). Hantaan virus infection, also known as Korean hemorrhagic fever or epidemic hemorrhagic fever, is the most common human disease due to hantaviruses. It was described before WW II in Manchuria along the Amur River, among United Nations troops during the Korean conflict, and subsequently in Japan, China, and in the Russian Far East. Severe disease from other hantaviruses also occurs in some Balkan states, including Bosnia, Serbia, and Greece. *Nephropathia epidemica*, a milder disease that occurs in Scandinavia and other parts of Europe, is caused by the Puumala virus carried by bank voles (small rodents of the genus *Microtus* and related genera). New World hantaviruses (i.e., Sin Nombre virus, Andes virus) cause hantavirus pulmonary syndrome (HPS) in the Americas. However, HPS generally leads to respiratory and cardiovascular failure rather than hemorrhagic fever.

Like the arenaviruses, hantaviruses are most commonly transmitted to humans via inhalation of dusts contaminated with rodent excreta.

Filoviridae: Four species of Ebola virus (Zaire, Sudan, Reston, Ivory Coast) and a new proposed species (Bundibugyo) have been identified. The Zaire and Sudan species of Ebola virus cause severe disease with high CFRs. Ebola hemorrhagic fever was first recognized in the western equatorial province of the Sudan (Ebola-Sudan) and a nearby region of Zaire (Ebola-Zaire) in 1976. In 1995 a single index case resulted in a large outbreak (316 cases) in Kikwit, Zaire. Subsequent epidemics of Ebola-Zaire and Sudan have occurred in Gabon, Ivory Coast, Uganda, Democratic Republic of Congo (former Zaire), and Sudan. The last reported Ebola-Zaire epidemic was in the DRC in 2007. Ebola-Reston was isolated from monkeys imported into the United States from the Philippine Islands in 1989. Infected monkeys developed hemorrhagic fever. There have been several outbreaks in non-human primate facilities since. In numerous cases, animal handlers have seroconverted, but did not manifest clinical disease. Therefore, Ebola-Reston has not been recognized as a human pathogen. In 2008, pigs were identified in the Philippines to be co-infected with Ebola-Reston and a porcine-specific virus. Some pig handlers seroconverted without clinical disease. The role of pigs, if any, in the natural ecology of this disease remains to be elucidated. In 1994, chimpanzees with lesions similar to those seen in humans infected with Ebola virus during the 1976 Ebola outbreaks were identified in the Tai Forest in Côte d'Ivoire, Africa. A scientist contracted the laboratory-confirmed Ebola-Ivory Coast virus after working with postmortem tissues and became ill. She made a full recovery. In 2007, a VHF outbreak occurred in Bundibugyo District in western Uganda (149 cases, 25% CFR). Laboratory analysis confirmed the newest and fifth species of Ebola virus. Recent data implicate bats as the likely reservoir, although the initial mode of spread to humans and the ecology of these disease remains to be worked out. It is not known why this disease appears intermittently. Unlike Ebola virus, only one species of Marburg virus (Lake Victoria) has been recognized. The first recognized outbreak occurred in Marburg, Germany and in Yugoslavia, among people exposed to African green monkeys in 1967. It resulted in 31 cases with seven deaths. Since 1967, Marburg epidemics have been sporadic and mostly in Africa. In 2005, an outbreak in Angola resulted in 324 deaths with a large percentage of fatalities seen in children. The Egyptian fruit bat (*Rousettus aegyptiacus*), found throughout Africa, is thought to be the reservoir for Marburg virus. Filoviruses may be spread from human to human by direct contact with infected blood, secretions, organs, or semen. Although frequently considered possible, spread from human to human by the airborne route occurs rarely, if it occurs at all. Ebola-Reston apparently spread from monkey to monkey and from monkeys to humans by the respiratory route.

Flaviviridae: Yellow fever and dengue are two mosquito-borne viruses that have great importance in the history of military campaigns and military medicine. Tick-borne flaviruses include the agents of Kyasanur Forest disease in India, and Omsk hemorrhagic fever in Siberia.

All of the VHF agents (except for dengue virus) are laboratory infectious hazards by aerosol, although even dengue has been nosocomially transmitted by blood splash. The aerosol infectivity for many VHF agents has been studied and measured in experimental animal models. VHF agents cause severe disease, and many have extremely high fatality rates. For these reasons, the VHF agents are considered a significant potential threat for biowarfare use.

CLINICAL FEATURES

Hemorrhagic fever viruses can lead to illnesses with diverse clinical presentations. In their most severe form, these diseases manifest as the "VHF syndrome", with capillary leak, bleeding diathesis, and hemodynamic compromise leading to shock. Early symptoms of VHF are nondescript in most cases, consisting of fever and constitutional symptoms such as malaise, myalgias, and headache. This constellation of findings is difficult to discern from any number of viral, bacterial, or parasitic diseases.

Diversity of clinical features among the VHFs probably stems from varying mechanisms of pathogenesis. For example, an immunopathogenic mechanism has been identified for dengue hemorrhagic fever, which usually occurs among patients previously infected with a heterologous dengue serotype. A prominent theory explaining this phenomenon is called "antibody-dependent enhancement." Disseminated intravascular coagulation (DIC) is thought to underlie the hemorrhagic features of Rift Valley, Marburg, and Ebola fevers; but in most VHFs, the etiology of the coagulopathy is multifactorial (e.g., hepatic damage, consumptive coagulopathy, and primary marrow dysfunction).

Why some infected persons develop full-blown VHF while others do not remains an unresolved issue. Virulence of the infecting agent clearly plays a large role. The VHF syndrome occurs in a majority of patients manifesting disease from filoviruses, CCHF, and the South American hemorrhagic fever viruses, while it occurs in a small minority of patients with dengue, RVF, and Lassa fever. The reasons for variation among patients infected with the same virus are still unknown but probably stem from a complex system of virus-host interactions.

Differentiating the various VHFs before laboratory diagnosis may be difficult. Epidemiological context may be helpful in this regard, especially discerning the proportion of cases with mild or moderate disease as compared to the proportion with severe disease, or knowledge of recent travel to known endemic areas. Astute clinicians who are familiar with the clinical presentations of the various VHF diseases may be able to pick out unique features that implicate one disease over the others. Clinical manifestations of the various VHFs are discussed below. Table 1 provides a summary of disease characteristics.

Arenaviridae: The clinical features of the South American hemorrhagic fevers (SAHFs) are quite similar, but they differ significantly from those of Lassa fever. Onset of the SAHFs is insidious, resulting in high unremitting fever and constitutional symptoms. A petechial or vesicular enanthem involving the palate and tonsillar pillars is quite common, as is conjunctival injection and flushing of the upper torso and face. Patients frequently have associated neurologic disease, with initial hyporeflexia followed by gait abnormalities and cerebellar dysfunction. Seizures portend a grave prognosis. Fatality rates from the SAHFs are high, ranging from 15% to over 30%.

By contrast, most natural infections with Lassa virus are mild or nonapparent. Less than 10% of infections result in severe disease, but fatality can be as high as 25%. Hemorrhagic phenomena are relatively uncommon, but patients frequently have retrosternal chest pain, sore throat and proteinuria. Syndromes with features of encephalitis and/or meningitis are sometimes present, as are convalescent cerebellar syndromes. Serum AST levels of 115 U/L or greater indicate a poor prognosis – this is often considered a criterion for treatment. Eighth nerve deafness is a common feature of Lassa fever. It occurs in the second or third week of illness and may be permanent. Transient alopecia is not uncommon during convalescence.

Bunyaviridae: CCHF is generally a severe, hemorrhagic disease. Onset is abrupt and GI and meningeal symptoms occur frequently. Petechiae and ecchymoses are common, as is mucosal bleeding. Hepatitis and jaundice probably results from direct viral cytotoxicity. Thrombocytopenia can be profound. CFR ranges from 20% to 50%.

RVF is usually a self-limited, nondescript febrile illness. About 10% of patients develop retinitis with cotton-wool exudates in or around the macula. This may result in permanent vision loss. Only 1% develop hemorrhagic manifestations or severe hepatic disease, usually occurring as a second febrile phase after defervescence from an initial febrile phase of 3–7 days. A small minority of patients develop encephalitis after the initial febrile illness.

The severity of hemorrhagic fever with renal syndrome (HFRS) depends largely on the infecting hantavirus. Puumala virus, common in northern Europe and Russia, causes a relatively mild form of disease (*nephropathica endemica*) that is associated with rare mortality. The most severe form of HFRS is caused by Hantaan virus. There are four clinical phases. In the initial febrile phase, disease onset is usually abrupt and is associated with fever, malaise, myalgia, headache, and lassitude. Some characteristic features are flushing of the face and neck, conjunctival and pharyngeal injection, cutaneous and mucosal petechiae (occurring by day 4 or 5), and profound lower back pain. In the second, hypotensive phase, mild DIC, thrombocytopenia, and capillary leak syndrome may ensue leading to hypovolemic shock. In the oliguric phase, renal dysfunction is pathognomonic, frequently progressing to oliguric renal failure. The final diuretic phase often accompanies convalescence, and fluid management may be a significant challenge. Death occurs in 5% to 15% of Hantaan infections.

Filoviridae: Ebola and Marburg infections present similarly. Onset is abrupt with fever, constitutional symptoms, nausea, vomiting, diarrhea, abdominal pain, lymphadenopathy, pharyngitis, conjuctival injection, and pancreatitis. A large number of patients develop a maculopapular rash around day 5, but this may be difficult to appreciate in dark-skinned persons. Elevated liver enzymes, increased blood urea nitrogen and creatinine, increased clotting times, and elevated d-dimers, but decreased fibrinogen are typical clinical pathology findings. Delirium, obtundation, and coma are common. Hemorrhagic features develop as the disease progresses. Death occurs at the beginning of the second week of illness. Fatality rates from 25% (Bundibugyo) to over 80% (Marburg/Ebola Zaire).

Flaviviridae: Yellow fever is classically described as a severe biphasic illness, but it is apparent that a large number of infections are mild or

TABLE 1: Comparison of VHF agents and diseases

	Virus	Disease	Endemic area	Fatality
Flavivirus	Yellow fever virus	Yellow fever	Africa, South America	Overall 3-12%, 20-50% if severe second phase develops
	KFD virus	Kyasanur Forest disease	Southern India	3-5%
	OHF virus	Omsk hemorrhagic fever	Siberia	0.2-3%
Filoviruses	Ebola virus	Ebola hemorrhagic fever	Africa, Philippines (Ebola Reston)	50-90% for Sudan/Zaire
	Marburg virus	Marburg hemor-rhagic fever	Africa	23-70%
Bunyaviruses	CCHF	Crimean-Congo hemorrhagic fever	Africa, SE Europe, Central Asia, India	30%
	RVF	Rift valley fever	Africa	<0.5%
	Hantavirus (Hantaan, Dobrava, Seoul, Puumala)	Hemorrhagic fever with renal syndrome (HFRS)	Europe, Asia, South America (rare)	5% for Asian HFRS
Arenaviruses	Lassa virus	Lassa fever	West Africa	1-2%
	Junin	Argentine hemorrhagic fever	Argentinean pampas	30%
	Machupo	Bolivian hemorrhagic	Bolivia	25-35%

Nosocomial transmission	Characteristic features	Countermeasures
No	Often biphasic, severe second phase with bleeding, very high bilirubin and transaminases, jaundice, renal failure	17-D live attenuated vaccine very effective in prevention, no postexposure countermeasure available
No	Flu-like syndrome with addition of cough, GI symptoms, hemorrhage, bradycardia	Formalin-inactivated vaccine available in India
No	Frequent sequelae of hearing loss, neuropsych complaints, alopecia	TBE vaccines (not avail. in US) may offer some cross-protection
Common	Severe illness, maculopapular rash, profuse bleeding and DIC	Anecdotal success with immune serum transfusion
Yes		
Yes	Often prominent petechial/ecchymotic rash	Anecdotal success with ribavirin
No	Hemorrhagic disease rare, classically associated with retinitis and encephalitis, Significant threat to livestock – epidemics of abortion and death of young	Effective livestock vaccines in Africa Human killed vaccine – DOD IND, live attenuated vaccine in clinical trials
No	Prominent renal disease, marked polyuric phase during recovery, usually elevated WBC	Effective locally produced vaccines in Asia (not avail in U.S.). Experimental vaccine at USAMRIID. Ribavirin effective in randomized, controlled clinical trial
Yes	Frequent unapparent/mild infection, hearing loss in convalescence common	Ribavirin effective in clinical trial with non-randomized controls
Rare	Prominent GI complaints, late neurologic syndrome	Immune plasma, Ribavirin effective Candid 1 vaccine protective but not avail. in U.S.
Rare	Similar to AHF	Immune plasma effective, ribavirin probably effective, Candid 1 vaccine protects monkeys

subclinical. The initial phase of illness lasts about 1 week and consists of fever, constitutional symptoms, GI symptoms and other undifferentiated symptoms. Objective findings are unimpressive except for the frequent appearance of relative bradycardia (Faget's sign) and leukopenia. Facial flushing and conjuctival injection may also be present. After a period of clinical improvement and defervescence (hours to days) some patients develop a second febrile phase. This so called period of intoxication is characterized by high fever, severe constitutional symptoms, obtundation, skin and mucous membrane hemorrhages, severe hepatitis and profound jaundice. Liver enzyme elevation occurs in a pattern consistent with hepatocellular damage, and bilirubin may be quite high. Proteinuria is almost universal and is an excellent diagnostic clue. As severe disease progresses, renal failure consistent with hepatorenal syndrome may ensue. Death occurs in 50% of patients with the hemorrhagic form of yellow fever.

The two members of the tick-borne encephalitis complex causing hemorrhagic disease (Kyasanur Forest and Omsk) have similar clinical syndromes and are often biphasic. The first phase is a febrile syndrome of varying severity, associated with conjunctival suffusion, facial flushing, lymphadenopathy, and splenomegaly. In its most severe form, this syndrome may be accompanied by diffuse mucosal hemorrhaging and petechiae. Hemorrhagic pulmonary edema is a relatively common and distinct feature. A second phase of illness may occur 1-3 wks after remission. This second phase involves mainly neurologic disease. Fatality ranges from < 3% (Omsk) up to 10% (Kyasanur Forest). Survivors may experience complications of iritis, keratitis, or neuropsychiatric abnormalities.

Dengue virus has not typically been considered a potential biological weapon agent, as it has not been shown in the laboratory to infect by aerosol. However, blood splashes in hospitals have spread the disease.

DIAGNOSIS

A VHF should be considered in any patient presenting with a severe, acute febrile illness and evidence of vascular instability (postural hypotension, petechiae, easy bleeding, flushing of face and chest, non-dependent edema). Symptoms and signs suggesting additional organ system involvement are common (headache, photophobia, pharyngitis, cough, nausea or vomiting, diarrhea, constipation, abdominal pain, hyperesthesia, dizziness, confusion, tremor) but usually do not dominate the picture, with the exceptions listed above under "Clinical Features." A positive tourniquet test has been particularly useful in dengue hemorrhagic fever, but should be sought in other hemorrhagic fevers as well.

A detailed travel history and a high index of suspicion are essential in making the diagnosis of VHF. Patients with arenavirus or hantavirus infections often recall proximity to rodents or their droppings; but as the viruses are spread to humans by aerosolized excreta or environmental contamination, direct contact with the infected rodents is not necessary. Large mosquito populations are common during RVF, yellow fever, or dengue transmission, but a history of mosquito bite is too common to be of diagnostic significance. Tick bites or nosocomial exposure are of some significance in suspecting CCHF. Large numbers of military personnel presenting with VHF manifestations in the same geographic area over a short time period should be considered a "red flag." A large natural outbreak is possible in an endemic setting, but a large number of cases should also prompt concern of a biowarfare attack.

The clinical laboratory can be very helpful in presumptive diagnosis of VHF. Thrombocytopenia (exception: Lassa) and leukopenia (exceptions: Lassa, Hantaan, and CCHF) are the rule. Proteinuria and/or hematuria are common, and their presence is characteristic of AHF, BHF, and HFRS. High AST elevation is nonspecific for, but correlates with, severity of Lassa fever, and jaundice is a poor prognostic sign in yellow fever. Higher viral loads, renal failure, a high AST/ALT ratio (7-12 times higher AST), and low calcium (<6 mg/dl) appear to be poor prognostic factors for filoviral disease.

In most geographic areas, the major consideration in the differential diagnosis is malaria. Bear in mind that parasitemia alone in patients partially immune to malaria does not prove that symptoms are due to malaria. Other diseases in the differential diagnosis should include typhoid fever, non-typhoidal salmonellosis, leptospirosis, rickettsial infections, shigellosis, relapsing fever, fulminant hepatitis, and meningococcemia. Non-infectious illnesses that could mimic VHF include acute leukemia, lupus erythematosus, idiopathic or thrombotic thrombocytopenic purpura, hemolytic uremic syndrome, and the multiple causes of DIC.

Definitive diagnosis in an individual case rests on specific virology diagnosis. Most patients have readily detectable viremia at presentation (exception: hantavirus infections). Rapid enzyme immunoassays can detect viral antigens in acute sera from patients with AHF, Lassa fever, RVF, CCHF, and yellow fever. Lassa- and Hantaan-specific IgM often are detectable during the acute illness. Lack of IgM response in filoviral infection is a poor prognostic sign. Diagnosis by virus replication and identification requires 3 to 10 d or longer. PCR assays have been developed at USAMRIID and the CDC, and they may be helpful in making a presumptive diagnosis. With the exception of dengue, specialized microbiological containment is required for safe handling of these viruses. Appropriate precautions should be observed in collection, handling, shipping, and processing of diagnostic samples. Both the CDC (Atlanta, Georgia) and USAMRIID (Frederick, Maryland) have diagnostic laboratories functioning at the highest (BSL-4 or P-4) containment level.

MEDICAL MANAGEMENT

General principles of supportive care apply to managing the hemodynamic, hematologic, pulmonary, and neurologic dimensions of VHF, regardless of the specific etiologic agent. Intensive care is required for the most severely ill patients. Healthcare providers employing vigorous fluid resuscitation of hypotensive patients must be mindful of the propensity of some VHFs (e.g., HFRS) for pulmonary capillary leak. Vasoactive or inotropic agents are frequently required. The benefits of intravascular devices and invasive hemodynamic monitoring must be carefully weighed against the significant risk of hemorrhage. Restlessness, confusion, myalgia, and hyperesthesia should be managed by conservative measures, including the judicious use of sedatives and analgesics. Mechanical ventilation, renal dialysis, and anti-seizure therapy may be required. Secondary infections may occur as with any patient managed with invasive procedures and devices.

Management of the hemorrhagic component of VHFs mirrors that for any patient with a systemic coagulopathy. Red blood cells, platelets, and clotting factors should be replaced, guided by clinical indication and coagulation parameters. Intramuscular injections, aspirin, and other anticoagulant drugs should be avoided. Steroids are not indicated.

The antiviral drug ribavirin is available for therapy of Lassa fever, HFRS, and CCHF under an IND protocol. A controlled clinical trial has clearly indicated that parenteral ribavirin reduces morbidity in HFRS. Several trials have suggested that ribavirin lowers both the morbidity and mortality of Lassa fever. In the HFRS field trials, treatment was effective if begun within the first 4 d of fever, and continued for a 10 d course. Both the CDC and DOD (USAMRIID) have IND protocols for the treatment of VHFs with IV ribavirin. Because the supply of IV ribavirin is limited, oral ribavirin may be required in a mass-casualty situation. Oral ribavirin is licensed for the treatment of hepatitis C infection and is commercially available in the United States. Because it is not approved for use in VHF, it should be used under an IND protocol if possible. Dosing recommendations for IV and oral ribavirin are included in Table 2. Side effects of ribavirin include modest reversible hemolytic anemia and bone marrow suppression. Ribavirin is teratogenic in laboratory animals, but no human data exist. Potential risks to the fetus must be weighed against the potential life-saving benefit in pregnant women with grave illness due to one of these VHFs. Safety in infants and children has not been established for IV ribavirin, but inhaled ribavirin has been used extensively in the treatment of respiratory syncytial virus infection in infants. Ribavirin has poor *in vitro* and *in vivo* activity against the filoviruses (Ebola and Marburg) and the flaviviruses (dengue, yellow fever, Omsk hemorrhagic fever and Kyanasur Forest disease).

AHF responds to therapy with two or more units of convalescent plasma containing adequate amounts of neutralizing antibody and given within 8 d of onset. BHF appears to respond to passive immune therapy as well. Convalescent serum or immune globulin for SAHFs is not readily available in the United States. This therapy is investigational and should be given only in consultation with experts.

PROPHYLAXIS

The 17D live attenuated yellow fever vaccine is the only licensed vaccine available for any of the hemorrhagic fever viruses. The Candid 1 vaccine for AHF is a live, attenuated, investigational vaccine developed at USAMRIID. It was highly efficacious in a randomized, controlled trial in

TABLE 2: Recommended ribavirin dosing for treatment of viral hemorrhagic fevers* (from Borio et al. JAMA; 287:2391-2405. 2002.)

		Intravenous	Oral
Adults	Loading dose	30 mg/kg IV (max 2 gm) once	2000 mg PO once
	Maintenance dose	16 mg/kg IV (max 1 gm) q6 h for 4 d	Wt > 75 kg: 600 mg PO bid for 10 d
		8 mg/kg IV (max 500 mg) q8 h for 6 d	Wt < 75 kg: 400 mg PO in AM, 600 mg PO in PM for 10 d
Children	Loading dose	Same as adult	30 mg/kg PO once
	Maintenance dose	Same as adult	7.5 mg/kg PO bid for 10 d

*for confirmed or suspected arenavirus or bunyavirus or VHF of unknown etiology

Argentine agricultural workers, and it appears to protect against BHF in non-human primates. Unfortunately, Candid 1 is no longer manufactured and is not available in the U.S. Both inactivated and live-attenuated RVF vaccines are currently under investigation. The inactivated version still is administered to at-risk laboratory workers. There are presently no vaccines for the other VHF agents available for human use in the United States. Several local vaccines for Omsk, Kyasanur Forest, HFRS and CCHF are used in endemic areas, but they have not been rigorously studied.

Persons with percutaneous or mucocutaneous exposure to blood, body fluids, secretions, or excretions from a patient with suspected VHF should immediately wash the exposed skin surfaces with soap and water and irrigate mucous membranes with copious amounts of water or saline.

Close personal contacts or anyone, including medical personnel, exposed to blood or secretions from VHF patients (particularly Lassa fever, CCHF, and filoviral diseases) should be monitored for symptoms, fever, and other signs during the established incubation period. After a presumed biowarfare attack with an unknown VHF virus, any fever of 101°F or greater should prompt evaluation and consideration for immediate treatment with IV ribavirin until the particular agent is determined. However, the utility of postexposure, pre-symptomatic ribavirin prophylaxis is questionable. The DOD IND protocol for ribavirin therapy of CCHF and Lassa fever may allow for prophylactic treatment of exposed personnel, in consultation with protocol investigators. Most patients will tolerate this regimen well, but should be under surveillance for breakthrough disease (especially after drug cessation) or adverse drug effects (principally anemia).

ISOLATION AND CONTAINMENT

These viruses pose special challenges for hospital infection control. With the exception of dengue and hantaviruses, VHF patients harbor significant levels of potentially infectious virus in blood, body fluids, or secretions. Special caution must be exercised in handling hypodermic needles and other sharps that could result in parenteral exposure. Strict adherence to VHF-specific barrier precautions will prevent nosocomial transmission in most cases.

Lassa, CCHF, Ebola, and Marburg viruses may be particularly prone to nosocomial spread due to periods of high viremia corresponding with bleeding propensity. In several instances, secondary infections among contacts and medical personnel without direct body fluid exposure have been documented. These instances have prompted concern of a rare phenomenon of aerosol transmission of infection. Therefore, when VHF is suspected, additional infection control measures are indicated. The patient should be hospitalized in a private room with an adjoining anteroom to be used for donning and removing protective barriers, storage of supplies, and decontamination of laboratory specimen containers. A negative-pressure isolation room with 6–12 air exchanges per h is ideal for all VHF patients and is strongly advised for patients with significant cough, hemorrhage, or diarrhea. All persons entering the room should wear double gloves, impermeable gowns with leg and shoe coverings (contact isolation), eye protection and HEPA (N-95) masks or positive-pressure air-purifying respirators (PAPRs). Note that though, that aerosol transmission person-to-person, if it occurs, is a rare occurrence.

In the absence of a large, fixed medical-treatment facility, or in the event of an overwhelming number of casualties, isolation rooms may not be available for all casualties. At a minimum, VHF patients should stay together in a separate building or in a ward with an air-handling system separate from the rest of the building when feasible. Access should be restricted to those personnel required to care for the patients. Personnel should wear contact and respiratory protection while in this patient-care area. Personnel should undergo an external decontamination procedure at the point of leaving the contaminated patient-care area. A building, room or designated area that is separated from the patient-care area should be established for donning and removing protective gear. All waste (including linens) leaving the patient-care area should be decontaminated with bleach or quaternary ammonium compounds and double-bagged in clearly labeled biohazard waste bags. Ideally, this waste will be incinerated or autoclaved.

Laboratory specimens should be double-bagged, and the exterior of the outer bag should be decontaminated before transport to the laboratory. Excreta and other contaminated materials should be autoclaved, or decontaminated by the liberal application of appropriate disinfectants. Clinical laboratory personnel are at significant risk for exposure and should employ a biosafety cabinet (if available) with barrier and respiratory precautions when handling specimens. Clinical specimens should be handled in a designated, isolated space within the lab. Access to this space should be limited and thorough decontamination of the space and equipment should be routine.

No carrier state has been observed for any VHF, but excretion of virus in urine or semen may occur for some time during convalescence. Survivors should avoid sexual contact for at least 3 months. In fatal cases, there should be minimal handling of the remains, which should ideally be sealed in leak-proof material for prompt burial or cremation.

BIOLOGICAL TOXINS

Toxins are harmful substances produced by living organisms (animals, plants, or microbes). They can be distinguished from chemical agents, such as VX, cyanide, or mustard by the following characteristics: they are not man-made, are non-volatile (no vapor hazard), are usually not dermally active (mycotoxins are the exception), and may be much more toxic (based on weight) than chemical agents. A toxin's lack of volatility is an important property as it makes it unlikely to produce either secondary or person-to-person exposures, or a persistent environmental hazard.

A toxin's utility as an aerosol weapon is determined by its magnitude of toxicity, stability, and ease of production. The bacterial toxins, such as botulinum toxins, are the most toxic substances (by weight) known (Appendix I). Less toxic compounds, such as the mycotoxins, are thousands of times less toxic than botulinum toxins, and have limited aerosol potential. The relationship between aerosol toxicity and the quantity of toxin required for an effective open-air exposure is shown in Appendix J, which demonstrates that for some agents such as the mycotoxins and ricin, very large (ton) quantities would be needed for an effective open-air attack in a dispersed tactical environment. Stability limits the open-air potential of some toxins. For example, botulinum and tetanus toxins are large-molecular-weight proteins that are easily denatured by environmental factors (heat, desiccation, or ultraviolet light), thus posing limited downwind threat. However, one important consideration is that some toxins (e.g., certain botulinum serotypes) may be effective terrorist weapons when delivered by contamination of the food supply. Finally, some toxins (e.g., saxitoxin), might be both stable and highly toxic, but are so difficult to extract from natural sources, that they can only feasibly be produced in minute quantities.

As with all biological weapons, potential to cause incapacitation as well as lethality must be considered. Depending on the goals of an adversary, incapacitating agents may be more effective than lethal agents. Large numbers of ill patients might overwhelm the medical and evacuation infrastructure, will require specific medical treatment not normally available in hospitals on a large scale (e.g., ventilator assistance), and will assuredly create panic and disruption among the affected population. Several toxins, such as staphylococcal enteroxin B (SEB), pose a significant incapacitating threat by causing illness at doses much lower than those required for lethality.

The four toxins considered most likely to be used as bio-agents are botulinum toxins, ricin, SEB, and T-2 mycotoxins.

Botulinum

SUMMARY

Signs and Symptoms: Symptoms usually begin with descending paralysis, manifested through cranial nerve palsies, including ptosis ("drooping eyelid"), blurred vision, diplopia (double vision), dry mouth and throat, dysphagia (difficulty swallowing), and dysphonia (voice impairment). These findings are followed by symmetrical descending flaccid paralysis, with generalized weakness and progression to respiratory failure. Symptoms are dose-dependent, may begin as early as 12-36 h after inhalation, but can take several days to develop after exposure to low doses of toxin.

Diagnosis: Primarily clinical. Bio-agent attack should be suspected if multiple casualties simultaneously present with progressive descending flaccid paralysis. Laboratory confirmation can be obtained by bioassay (mouse neutralization) of the patient's serum. This bioassay is the accepted "gold standard" and widely used method for detecting botulinum neurotoxin (BoNT), but can take up to 4 d for completion. Nerve conduction studies and electromyography can prove useful in the differential diagnosis. Other assays that may be used for environmental or clinical samples, but lack formal accreditation and/or standardization, include ELISA or electrochemiluminescence (ECL) for bacterial antigen, polymerase chain reaction (PCR) for bacterial DNA, and reverse transcriptase-PCR (RT-PCR) for mRNA to detect active synthesis of toxin.

Treatment: Early administration of heptavalent antitoxin (an IND product) may prevent or decrease progression to respiratory failure and hasten recovery. Intubation and ventilatory assistance are needed for respiratory failure. Tracheostomy may be required for long-term airway maintenance.

Prophylaxis: Pentavalent toxoid vaccine (potential protection for types A, B, C, D, and E; but not F or G) is available as an IND product for those at high risk of exposure. It should be noted that, since the original toxoid components were produced in 1970, a decline in potency has been observed to some of the toxin serotypes (serotypes C, D, and E with the currently used pentavalent toxoid lot).

Isolation and Decontamination: Standard precautions are recommended for healthcare workers. BoNT is not dermally active and secondary aerosols are not a hazard from patients. Decontaminate with soap and water. BoNT is inactivated by sunlight within 1-3 h. Heat (80°C for 30 min, 100°C for several min) and chlorine (>99.7% inactivation by 3 mg/L free available chlorine (FAC) in 20 min) also destroy BoNT.

OVERVIEW

The BoNTs are a group of seven related neurotoxins produced by the spore-forming bacillus *Clostridium botulinum* (Types A through G) and three other *Clostridum* species (*C. butyricum* [Type E], *C. baratii* [Type F], and *C. argentinense* [Type G]). These toxins are the most potent neurotoxins known; paradoxically, they have been used therapeutically to treat spastic conditions (strabismus, blepharospasm, torticollis, tetanus) and cosmetically to efface wrinkles. The spores are ubiquitous; they germinate into vegetative bacteria that produce toxins during anaerobic incubation. Industrial-scale fermentation can potentially produce large quantities of toxin for use as a bio-agent. There are three epidemiologic forms of naturally occurring botulism - foodborne, intestinal (infant or adult intestinal), and wound botulism. Botulinum toxin could be delivered via aerosol or used to contaminate food or water supplies. When inhaled, these toxins produce a clinical picture very similar to foodborne intoxication. The clinical syndrome (regardless of epidemiological form of disease) produced by these toxins is known as "botulism." Natural human botulism is primarily caused by BoNT A, B, and E.

HISTORY AND SIGNIFICANCE

BoNTs have caused numerous cases of botulism when ingested in improperly prepared or canned foods. Many deaths have occurred from such incidents. It is theoretically possible, although difficult, to deliver BoNTs as an aerosolized biological weapon. Several countries and terrorist groups have weaponized BoNTs. BoNTs were weaponized by the U.S. in its now defunct offensive biowarfare program. Evidence obtained by the United Nations in 1995 revealed that Iraq had filled and deployed over 100 munitions with nearly 10,000 liters of botulinum toxin. The Aum Shinrikyo cult in Japan sought to weaponize and disseminate botulinum toxin on multiple occasions in Tokyo. After failing in these attempts, they then undertook a sarin attack in the Tokyo subway.

TOXIN CHARACTERISTICS

BoNTs are proteins with a molecular mass of approximately 150,000 daltons. Each of the seven toxin serotypes act to inhibit presynaptic acetylcholine release. The toxins produce similar effects when inhaled or ingested, although the time course may vary depending on the route of exposure and the dose received. BoNT could be used to sabotage food supplies, as has been theorized in the scientific literature.

These large proteins are readily denatured by environmental conditions. They are detoxified in open air within 12 h. Sunlight inactivates the toxins within 1-3 h. Heat destroys the toxins in 30 min at 80°C and in several min at 100°C. In water, the toxins are >99.7% inactivated by 20 min of exposure to 3 mg/L free available chlorine (FAC) similar to the military disinfection procedure; and 84% inactivated by 20 min at 0.4% mg/L FAC, similar to municipal water treatment procedures.

MECHANISM OF TOXICITY

BoNT consists of two polypeptide subunits (A and B chains). The B subunit binds to receptors on the axons of motor neurons. The toxin is taken into the axon, where the A chain exerts its cytotoxic effect; it inactivates the axon, preventing release of acetylcholine (ACh) and blocking neuromuscular transmission (pre-synaptic inhibition). Recovery follows only after the neuron develops a new axon, which can take months. The presynaptic inhibition affects both cholinergic autonomic (muscarinic) and motor (nicotinic) receptors. This interruption of neurotransmission may affect cranial nerves and nerves innervating skeletal muscle (resulting in paralysis) and the autonomic nervous system (nonreactive and dilated pupils, constipation, dry mouth, orthostatic hypotension).

Unlike the situation with nerve agent intoxication, where there is too much ACh due to inhibition of acetylcholinesterase, the problem in botulism is lack of the neurotransmitter in the synapse. Thus, pharmacologic measures such as atropine are not indicated in botulism and could exacerbate symptoms (see Appendix H).

CLINICAL FEATURES

The onset of symptoms of inhalation botulism usually occurs from 12 to 36 h after exposure, but can vary according to the amount of toxin absorbed and could be reduced following a biowarfarebiowarfare attack. Recent primate studies indicate that the signs and symptoms may not appear for several days when a low dose of the toxin is inhaled versus a shorter time period after ingestion of toxin or inhalation of higher doses.

Descending paralysis leads to cranial nerve palsies that are prominent early, with eye symptoms such as blurred vision due to mydriasis, diplopia, ptosis, and photophobia, in addition to other cranial nerve signs such as dysarthria, dysphonia, and dysphagia. Flaccid skeletal muscle paralysis follows, in a symmetrical, descending, and progressive manner. Collapse and obstruction of the upper airway may occur due to weakness of the oropharyngeal musculature. As the descending motor weakness involves the diaphragm and accessory muscles of respiration, respiratory failure may occur abruptly. Progression from onset of symptoms to respiratory failure has occurred in as little as 24 h in cases of severe food-borne botulism.

The autonomic effects of botulism are manifested by typical anticholinergic signs and symptoms: dry mouth, ileus, constipation, and urinary retention. Nausea and vomiting may occur as nonspecific sequelae of an ileus. Dilated pupils (mydriasis) are seen in approximately 50% of cases.

Sensory symptoms usually do not occur. BoNT do not cross the blood/brain barrier and do not cause CNS disease. However, the psychological sequelae of botulism may be severe and require specific intervention.

Physical examination usually reveals an afebrile, alert, and oriented patient, although the paralysis may limit the patient's ability to respond. Postural hypotension may be present. Mucous membranes may be dry and crusted and the patient may complain of dry mouth or sore throat. There may be difficulty with speaking and swallowing. Gag reflex may be absent. Pupils may be dilated and even fixed. Ptosis and extraocular muscle palsies may also be present. Variable degrees of skeletal muscle weakness may be observed depending on the degree of progression in an individual patient. Deep tendon reflexes may be diminished or absent. With severe respiratory muscle paralysis, the patient may become cyanotic or exhibit narcosis from CO_2 retention.

DIAGNOSIS

The occurrence of an epidemic of afebrile patients with progressive symmetrical descending flaccid paralysis would strongly suggest botulinum intoxication. Food-borne outbreaks have most often occurred in small clusters. Higher numbers of confirmed cases in a theater of operations should at least raise the consideration of a BoNT attack.

Individual cases might be confused clinically with other neuromuscular disorders such as Guillain-Barre syndrome, myasthenia gravis, or tick paralysis. The edrophonium or *Tensilon®* test may be transiently positive in botulism, so it may not distinguish botulinum intoxication from myasthenia. The CSF in botulism is normal and the paralysis is generally symmetrical, which distinguishes it from enteroviral myelitis. Mental status changes generally seen in viral encephalitis should not occur with botulinum intoxication.

It may become necessary to distinguish nerve agent and/or atropine poisoning from botulinum intoxication. Nerve agent poisoning produces copious respiratory secretions, miotic pupils, convulsions, and muscle twitching, whereas normal secretions, mydriasis, difficulty swallowing, and progressive muscle paralysis is more likely in botulinum intoxication. Atropine overdose is distinguished from botulism by its CNS excitation (hallucinations and delirium) even though the mucous membranes are dry and mydriasis is present. The clinical differences between botulinum intoxication and nerve agent poisoning are depicted in Appendix H.

Laboratory testing is generally not critical to the diagnosis of botulism. Botulism is foremost a clinical diagnosis, and laboratory results can be inconclusive. Mouse neutralization (bioassay) remains the most sensitive test available. Therefore, serum samples should be drawn and sent to a laboratory capable performing this assay. Other tests lack formal accreditation and/or standardization. PCR might detect *C. botulinum* genes in clinical specimens or environmental samples, but it must only be used in conjunction with the mouse bioassay, as PCR is not accredited for this purpose. Detecting toxin in clinical or environmental samples is sometimes possible by ELISA or ECL-based immunoassay. Clinical samples can include serum, gastric aspirates, stool, and respiratory secretions. Survivors do not usually develop an antibody response due to the very small amount of toxin necessary to produce clinical symptoms. Exposure does not confer immunity.

MEDICAL MANAGEMENT

Supportive care, including prompt respiratory support, can be lifesaving. Respiratory failure due to paralysis of respiratory muscles is the most serious effect and, generally, the cause of death. Botulism cases reported before 1950 had a case fatality rate (CFR) of 60%. With the intervention as appropriate of tracheotomy or endotracheal intubation, ventilatory assistance, coupled with administration of botulinum immunoglobulin, CFRs are less than 5% today. However, initially unrecognized cases may have a higher fatality. Preventing nosocomial infections is a primary concern, along with hydration, nasogastric suctioning for ileus, bowel and bladder care, and preventing decubitus ulcers and deep venous thromboses. Intensive and prolonged nursing care may be required for recovery, which may take up to 3 months for initial signs of improvement, and up to a year for complete resolution of symptoms.

Antitoxin: Early administration of botulinum antitoxin is critical, as the antitoxin neutralizes the circulating toxin in patients with symptoms that continue to progress. The antitoxin has no effect on toxin already bound to the nerve terminals. However, antitoxin is *never* withheld from the patient, even with delayed treatment.

Two different antitoxin preparations are available in the U.S. A bivalent human IV antiserum (types A and B, "BabyBIG") was licensed in October 2003 by the FDA and is available from the California Department of Health Services for treating infant botulism. This purified immunoglobulin is derived from pooled adult plasma from persons who were vaccinated with pentavalent botulinum toxoid and selected for their high titers of neutralizing antibody against botulinum neurotoxins type A and B.

A "despeciated" equine heptavalent antitoxin preparations against all seven serotypes has been prepared by cleaving the Fc fragments from horse IgG molecules, leaving $F(ab)_2$ fragments. The original product was developed by USAMRIID. As of March 13, 2010, an IND product -- *Heptavalent Botulinum AntiToxin* (*HBAT*, Cangene Corporation) -- became the only botulinum antitoxin available in the U.S. at the CDC for botulism. *Botulinum Antitoxin, Heptavalent, Equine, Types A, B, C, D, E, F, and G* (*HE-BAT*) is available to the military under IND protocols. Use of the equine antitoxin requires compliance with the IND protocol. Administration of equine antitoxins may first require skin testing with escalating dose challenges to assess the degree of an individual's sensitivity to horse serum before full-dose administration of the vaccine. Skin scratch tests should always precede intradermal tests. Skin testing is performed by injecting 0.1 ml of a 1:10 dilution (in sterile physiological saline) of antitoxin intradermally in the patient's forearm with a 26 or 27 gauge needle. The injection site is monitored and the patient is observed allergic reaction for 20 min. The skin test is positive if any of these allergic reactions occur: hyperemic areola at the site of the injection > 0.5 cm; fever or chills; hypotension with decrease of blood pressure > 20 mm Hg for systolic and diastolic pressures; skin rash; respiratory difficulty; nausea or vomiting; generalized itching. Equine-derived botulinum $F(ab')_2$ antitoxin is NOT administered if the skin test is positive. If no allergic symptoms are observed, the antitoxin is administered as a single IV dose in a normal saline solution, 10 ml over 20 min.

With a positive skin test, desensitization can be attempted by administering 0.01 - 0.1 ml of antitoxin subcutaneously, doubling the previous dose every 20 min until 1.0 - 2.0 ml can be sustained without any marked reaction. Ideally, desensitization would be performed by an experienced allergist. Medical personnel administering the HE-BAT antitoxin should be prepared to treat anaphylaxis with epinephrine, intubation equipment, and IV access.

PROPHYLAXIS

Vaccine: A pentavalent toxoid (PBT) of *C. botulinum* toxin types A, B, C, D, and E is available as an IND for preexposure prophylaxis. This product has been administered to several thousand volunteers and occupationally at-risk workers, and historically induced serum antitoxin levels that correspond to protective levels in experimental animals. At-risk laboratory workers remain the primary recipients. The PBT is currently given as a primary series of 0, 2, and 12 weeks, followed by a 6-month dose 1 yr booster. Previously, additional need for boosters was determined by antibody testing. Due to the decline in potency to some of the toxin serotypes, annual booster doses have been recommended since 2004. Laboratory workers are to consider personal protective measures to be the sole protection against botulinum toxin.

Contraindications to the vaccine include sensitivities to alum, formaldehyde, and thimerosal, or hypersensitivity to a previous dose. Systemic reactions are reported in up to 3%, consisting of fever, malaise, headache, and myalgia. Incapacitating reactions (local or systemic) are uncommon. More recent data based on active surveillance revealed 23% reported local reactions and 7.4% reported systemic reactions. The vaccine should be stored at 2-8°C (not frozen).

The vaccine is typically recommended for selected individuals or groups who work with the BoNTs in the laboratory. Because of the challenges of administering an IND product in an operational environment, and due to the concerns related to vaccine potency, only those individuals who have an extremely high risk of exposure to BoNTs in the field should be considered for receipt of the vaccine. There is no indication at present for using botulinum antitoxin as a prophylactic modality except under extremely specialized circumstances.

Postexposure prophylaxis, using a heptavalent antitoxin, has been demonstrated effective in animal studies; however, as human data are not available, it is generally not recommended. This usage of heptavalent antitoxin may be considered after a known high-risk exposure to BoNT had occurred (i.e., a high-risk laboratory exposure) for all exposed, as an extraordinary circumstance.

Ricin

SUMMARY

Signs and Symptoms: Fever, chest tightness, cough, dyspnea, nausea, and arthralgias occur 4 to 8 h after inhalational exposure. Airway necrosis and pulmonary capillary leak resulting in pulmonary edema may occur within 18-24 h, followed by severe respiratory distress and death from hypoxemia in 36-72 h.

Diagnosis: Acute lung injury in large numbers of geographically clustered patients may suggest exposure to aerosolized ricin. Nonspecific laboratory and radiographic findings include leukocytosis and bilateral interstitial infiltrates. The short time to severe symptoms and death would be unusual for infectious agents. Serum and respiratory secretions should be submitted for antigen detection by ELISA. Acute and convalescent sera allow retrospective diagnosis.

Treatment: Supportive; includes management of pulmonary edema. Gastric lavage and cathartics are indicated for ricin ingestion, but charcoal is of little value for such large molecules.

Prophylaxis: Using a mask is currently the best protection against inhalation. There is currently no licensed vaccine or prophylactic antitoxin available for human use. However, there are two IND vaccines in development. A mutant recombinant RTA, *RiVax*, has been shown to be safe and immunogenic in humans in a Phase 1 trial. A second clinical trial is being supported by FDA's Orphan Products Division. The second vaccine candidate is a recombinant ricin toxin A-chain (*RVEc*) which has shown promise in animal models. It will enter Phase 1 trials in 2011.

Isolation and Decontamination: Standard precautions are for healthcare workers. Ricin is non-volatile, and secondary aerosols are not expected to be a hazard. Decontaminate with soap and water. Hypochlorite solutions (0.1% sodium hypochlorite) inactivate ricin.

OVERVIEW

Ricin is a potent protein cytotoxin derived from the beans of the castor plant (*Ricinus communis*). Castor beans are ubiquitous worldwide, and the toxin is fairly easy to extract. Therefore, ricin is widely available. When inhaled as a small-particle aerosol, this toxin may produce pathologic changes within 8 h and severe respiratory symptoms followed by acute hypoxic respiratory failure in 36-72 h. When ingested, ricin causes severe gastrointestinal symptoms followed by vascular collapse and death. Intramuscular injection causes induration and necrosis locally and depending on dose may cause fever, nausea, vomiting, tachycardia, hypotension, leukocytosis, renal failure, hematemesis, liver failure, and cardiac arrest. This toxin also causes disseminated intravascular coagulation, microcirculatory failure, and multiple organ failure when given intravenously in laboratory animals.

HISTORY AND SIGNIFICANCE

Ricin toxin's significance as a potential bioagent relates in part to its wide availability. Worldwide, one million tons of castor beans are processed annually in the production of castor oil; the waste mash from this process is 3-5% ricin by weight. The toxin is also quite stable and extremely toxic by several routes of exposure, including the respiratory route. Ricin was apparently used in the assassination of Bulgarian exile Georgi Markov in London in 1978. Markov was attacked with a specially engineered weapon disguised as an umbrella, which implanted a ricin-containing pellet into his body. This technique was used in at least six other assassination attempts in the late 1970s and early 1980s. In 1994 and 1995, four men from a tax-protest group known as the "Minnesota Patriots Council," were convicted of possessing ricin and conspiring to use it (by mixing it with the solvent dimethylsulfoxide) to murder law enforcement officials. In 1995, a Kansas City oncologist, Deborah Green, attempted to murder her husband by ricin food contamination. In 1997, a Wisconsin resident, Thomas Leahy, was arrested and charged with possession with intent to use ricin as a weapon. In 2003, ricin powder was discovered in a South Carolina incident and in 2004 in the mail room of a United States senator. Laboratory analysis of samples from the South Carolina incident revealed no ricin contamination. No confirmed cases of ricin-associated illness were identified. Ricin has a high terrorist potential due to its ready availability, relative ease of extraction, and notoriety in the media.

TOXIN CHARACTERISTICS

Ricin consists of two hemagglutinins and two toxins. The toxins, RCL III and RCL IV, are dimers with molecular masses of about 66,000 daltons. The toxins are made up of two polypeptide chains, an A chain and a B chain, which are joined by a disulfide bond. Large quantities of ricin can be produced relatively easily and inexpensively by a simple technology. Ricin can be prepared in liquid or crystalline form, or it can be lyophilized to make a dry powder. It can be disseminated as an aerosol, injected into a victim, or used to contaminate food or water. Ricin is stable under typical ambient conditions, but is detoxified by heat (80°C for 10 min or 50°C for about an h at pH 7.8) and chlorine [>99.4% inactivation by 100 mg/L free available chlorine (FAC) in 20 min]. Low chlorine concentrations, such as 10 mg/L FAC, as well as iodine at up to 16 mg/L, have no effect on ricin. Ricin's toxicity (LD_{50}) is marginal compared to other toxins, such as botulinum and SEB (incapacitating dose). An enemy would need to produce it in large quantities to cover a significant area on the battlefield, limiting its utility.

MECHANISM OF TOXICITY

Ricin's cytotoxicity is due to inhibition of protein synthesis. The B chain binds to cell-surface receptors and the toxin-receptor complex is taken into the cell; the A chain has endonuclease activity and even very low concentrations will inhibit DNA replication and protein synthesis. In rodents, the histopathology of aerosol exposure is characterized by necrosis of upper and lower respiratory epithelium, causing tracheitis, bronchitis, bronchiolitis, and interstitial pneumonia with perivascular and alveolar edema. There is a latent period of 8 h after inhalation exposure before histologic lesions are observed in animal models. In rodents, ricin is more toxic by the aerosol route than by other routes.

CLINICAL FEATURES

The clinical picture depends on the route of exposure. After aerosol exposure, signs and symptoms depend on the dose inhaled. Accidental sublethal aerosol exposures, which occurred in humans in the 1940s, were characterized by onset of fever, chest tightness, cough, dyspnea, nausea, and arthralgias within 4 to 8 h. The onset of profuse sweating some hours later was commonly the sign of termination of most of the symptoms. Although lethal human aerosol exposures have not been described, the severe pathophysiologic changes seen in the animal respiratory tract, including necrosis and severe alveolar flooding, were sufficient to cause death from acute respiratory distress syndrome (ARDS) and respiratory failure. Time to death in experimental animals is dose dependent, occurring 36-72 h after inhalation. Exposed humans can be expected to develop severe lung inflammation with progressive cough, dyspnea, cyanosis, and pulmonary edema.

By other routes of exposure, ricin is not a direct lung irritant; however, intravascular injection can cause minimal pulmonary perivascular edema due to vascular endothelial injury. Ingestion causes necrosis of the GI epithelium, local hemorrhage, and hepatic, splenic, and renal necrosis. Intramuscular injection causes severe local necrosis of muscle and regional lymph nodes with moderate visceral organ involvement.

DIAGNOSIS

An attack with aerosolized ricin would be primarily diagnosed by the clinical features in the appropriate epidemiological context. Acute lung injury affecting a large number of geographically clustered cases should raise suspicion of an attack with a pulmonary irritant such as ricin, although other pulmonary pathogens could present with similar signs and symptoms. Other biological threats, such as SEB, Q fever, tularemia, plague, and some chemical warfare agents like phosgene, need to be included in the differential diagnosis. Ricin-induced pulmonary edema would be expected to occur much later (1-3 days postexposure) compared to that induced by SEB (about 12 h postexposure) or phosgene (about 6 h postexposure). Ricin intoxication will progress despite treatment with antibiotics, in contrast to an infectious process. Ricin intoxication does not cause mediastinitis as with inhalational anthrax. Ricin patients do not plateau clinically as with SEB intoxication. Additional supportive clinical or diagnostic features after aerosol exposure to ricin include the following: bilateral infiltrates on CXR, arterial hypoxemia, neutrophilic leukocytosis, and a bronchial aspirate rich in protein compared to plasma, which is characteristic of high-permeability pulmonary edema.

Specific ELISA and ECL tests of serum and respiratory secretions, or immunohistochemical stains of tissue may be used where available to confirm the diagnosis. Ricin is an extremely immunogenic toxin, and paired acute and convalescent sera should be obtained from survivors to measure antibody response. PCR can be used to detect castor bean DNA in most ricin preparations.

MEDICAL MANAGEMENT

Management of ricin-intoxicated patients differs depending on the exposure route. Patients with pulmonary intoxication are managed by appropriate level of respiratory support (oxygen, intubation, ventilation, positive end-expiratory pressure (PEEP), and hemodynamic monitoring) and treatment for pulmonary edema, as indicated. GI intoxication is best managed by vigorous gastric lavage, followed by use of cathartics, such as magnesium citrate. Superactivated charcoal administration to the patient is of little value for large molecules such as ricin. Volume replacement of GI fluid losses is important. In percutaneous exposures, treatment is primarily supportive.

PROPHYLAXIS

The M-40 protective mask is effective in preventing aerosol exposure. Although a vaccine is not currently available, candidate vaccines are under development. These are immunogenic and confer protection against lethal aerosol exposures in animals. Preexposure prophylaxis with such a vaccine is the most promising defense against a biowarfare attack with ricin.

Staphylococcal Enterotoxin B (SEB)

SUMMARY

Signs and Symptoms: A latent period of 3-12 h after aerosol exposure is followed by sudden onset of fever, chills, headache, myalgia, and nonproductive cough. Some patients may develop shortness of breath and retrosternal chest pain. Patient symptoms tend to plateau soon at a fairly stable clinical state. Fever may last 2 to 5 days, and cough may persist for up to 4 weeks. Patients may also present with nausea, vomiting, and diarrhea. GI symptoms are likely to be more profound if toxin is swallowed. Delivery of high doses will result in toxic shock and death.

Diagnosis: Clinical. Patients present with a febrile respiratory syndrome without CXR abnormalities. Large numbers of patients presenting in a short time with typical symptoms and signs of SEB aerosol exposure suggest an intentional attack with this toxin.

Treatment: Supportive. Artificial ventilation may be needed for very severe cases, and attention to fluid management is essential.

Prophylaxis: Protective mask. There is currently no human vaccine available.

Isolation and Decontamination: Standard precautions are recommended for healthcare workers. SEB is not dermally active and secondary aerosols are not a hazard. It can be decontaminated with soap and water and any contaminated food should be destroyed.

OVERVIEW

Staphylococcus aureus produces a number of exotoxins, one of which is staphylococcal enterotoxin B (SEB). Such toxins are referred to as exotoxins as they are excreted from the organism, and as they normally exert their effects on the intestines, they are known as enterotoxins. SEB is one of the pyrogenic toxins that commonly cause food poisoning in humans after the toxin is produced in improperly handled foodstuffs and subsequently ingested. SEB has a very broad spectrum of biological activity. This toxin causes markedly different clinical syndromes when inhaled versus ingested. Significant morbidity is produced by both portals of entry.

HISTORY AND SIGNIFICANCE

Staphylococcal enterotoxins like SEB are a common cause of food poisoning outbreaks. These often occur in a group setting such as a church picnic or other community event, and are due to improperly handled food and temperature holding, combined with a common-source exposure in which the contaminated food is consumed. Although an aerosolized SEB weapon would not likely produce significant mortality, it could render 80% or more of exposed personnel clinically ill and unable to perform their mission for 1-2 weeks. The resulting demand on medical and logistical systems could be overwhelming. For these reasons, SEB was one of the seven bio-agents stockpiled by the U.S. during its offensive bioweapons program (1943-1969).

TOXIN CHARACTERISTICS

Staphylococcal enterotoxins are proteins of 23-29 kilodaltons molecular mass (SEB is 28,494 daltons). They are extracellular products of coagulase-positive staphylococci. Up to 50% of clinical isolates of *S. aureus* produce exotoxins. They are produced in culture media and also in foods when there is overgrowth of the bacterium. Related toxins include toxic-shock syndrome toxin-1 (TSST-1) and exfoliative toxins. SEB is one of at least seven antigenically distinct enterotoxins that have been classically identified. These toxins are moderately stable; SEB is inactivated after a few min at 100°C. SEB causes symptoms when inhaled at even very low doses in humans: a dose of several logs lower (at least 100 times less) than the lethal dose by the inhaled route would be sufficient to incapacitate 50% of those exposed. This toxin could also be used to sabotage food or small-volume water supplies.

MECHANISM OF TOXICITY

Staphylococcal enterotoxins belong to a class of potent immune stimulants known as bacterial superantigens. Superantigens bind to major histocompatibility complex type II receptors on antigen-presenting cells, leading to the direct stimulation of large populations of T-helper cells while bypassing the usual antigen processing and presentation. This induces a brisk cascade of pro-inflammatory cytokines (such as tumor necrosis factor, interferon, interleukin-1 and interleukin-2), with recruitment of other immune effector cells, and relatively deficient activation of counter-regulatory negative feedback loops. This results in an intense inflammatory response that injures host tissues. Released cytokines are thought to mediate many of the toxic effects of SEB.

CLINICAL FEATURES

Symptoms of SEB intoxication begin after a latent period of 3-12 h after inhalation, or 4-10 h after ingestion. Initial symptoms after either route may include nonspecific flu-like symptoms such as fever, chills, headache, and myalgias. Subsequent symptoms depend upon the route of exposure. Ingestion results in predominantly GI symptoms: nausea, vomiting, and diarrhea. Inhalation produces predominantly respiratory symptoms: nonproductive cough, retrosternal chest pain, and dyspnea. GI symptoms may accompany respiratory exposure due to inadvertent swallowing of the toxin after normal mucocilliary clearance, or simply as a systemic manifestation of intoxication. GI symptoms have also been seen in ocular exposures in which ingestion was not thought to have occurred. Ocular exposure results in conjunctivitis with associated periorbital edema.

Respiratory pathology is due to the activation of pro-inflammatory cytokine cascades in the lungs, leading to pulmonary capillary leak and pulmonary edema. Severe cases may result in acute pulmonary edema and respiratory failure.

Fever may last up to 5 days and range from 103 to 106°F, with variable degrees of chills and prostration. Cough may persist for up to 4 weeks, and patients may not be able to return to duty for 2 weeks.

Physical examination in patients with SEB intoxication is often unremarkable. Conjunctival injection may be present, and postural hypotension may develop due to fluid losses. Chest examination is unremarkable except in the unusual case where pulmonary edema develops. CXR is usually normal, but in severe cases increased interstitial markings, atelectasis, and occasionally pulmonary edema or acute respiratory distress syndrome (ARDS) may develop.

DIAGNOSIS

Diagnosis of SEB intoxication is based on clinical and epidemiologic features. Because the symptoms of SEB intoxication may be similar to several respiratory pathogens including influenza, adenovirus, and mycoplasma, the diagnosis may initially be unclear. All of these illnesses might present with fever, nonproductive cough, myalgia, and headache. An SEB attack would cause cases to present in numbers over a very short time, probably within a single 24 h. Influenza or community-acquired pneumonia should involve patients presenting over a more prolonged interval. Naturally occurring staphylococcal food poisoning does not present with pulmonary symptoms. Symptoms of SEB intoxication tends to plateau rapidly to a fairly stable clinical state, whereas inhalational anthrax, tularemia pneumonia, or pneumonic plague would all continue to progress if left untreated. Tularemia and plague, as well as Q fever (all bacterial infections, unlike SEB intoxication), are often associated with infiltrates on chest radiographs. Other diseases, including hantavirus pulmonary syndrome, *Chlamydia* pneumonia, and various chemical warfare agents (mustard, phosgene via inhalation) are included in the initial differential diagnosis.

Laboratory confirmation of SEB intoxication includes antigen detection (ELISA, ECL) on environmental and clinical samples, and gene amplification (PCR – to detect staphylococcal genes) on environmental samples. SEB may not be detectable in the serum by the time symptoms occur; nevertheless, a serum specimen should be drawn as early as possible after exposure. Data from rabbit studies clearly show that the presence of SEB in the serum is transient; however, accumulation in the urine was detected for several hours postexposure in these animals (unpublished, USAMRIID). It may therefore prove useful to obtain urine samples for testing. Respiratory secretions and nasal swabs may demonstrate the toxin early (within 24 h of exposure). Because most patients develop a significant antibody response to the toxin, acute and convalescent sera should be drawn for retrospective diagnosis. Nonspecific findings include neutrophilic leukocytosis, elevated erythrocyte sedimentation rate, and CXR abnormalities consistent with pulmonary edema.

MEDICAL MANAGEMENT

Currently, therapy is limited to supportive care. Close attention to oxygenation and hydration is important, and in severe cases with pulmonary edema, ventilation with positive end-expiratory pressure, vasopressors and diuretics may be necessary. Acetaminophen for fever, and cough suppressants may make the patient more comfortable. The value of treatment with steroids is unknown. Most patients can be expected to do quite well after the initial acute phase of their illness, but will be unfit for duty for 1 to 2 weeks. Severe cases are at risk of death from pulmonary edema and respiratory failure.

PROPHYLAXIS

Although there is currently no human vaccine for SEB intoxication, several vaccine candidates are in development. Preliminary animal studies have been encouraging. A vaccine candidate is nearing transition to advanced development for safety and immunogenicity testing in humans. Experimentally, passive immunotherapy can reduce mortality in animals, but only when given within 4-8 h after inhalation. Because of the rapidity of SEB binding with MHC Class II receptors (<5 min *in vitro*), active vaccination is considered the most practical defense. Interestingly, most people have detectable baseline antibody titers to SEB; however, immunity acquired through natural exposure to SEB does not adequately protect against an aerosol challenge (although it may reduce the emetic effect).

T-2 Mycotoxins

SUMMARY

Signs and symptoms: Exposure causes skin pain, pruritus, redness, vesiculation, necrosis, and sloughing of the epidermis. Effects on the airway include nose and throat pain, nasal discharge, itching and sneezing, cough, dyspnea, wheezing, chest pain, and hemoptysis. Similar effects occur after ingestion or eye contact. Severe intoxication results in weakness, ataxia, collapse, prostration, shock, and death.

Diagnosis: The toxin should be suspected if an aerosol attack occurs in the form of "yellow rain" with droplets of variously pigmented oily fluids contaminating clothes and the environment. Confirmation requires testing of blood, tissue and environmental samples.

Treatment: No specific antidote; treatment is supportive. Soap and water washing, even 4-6 h after exposure, can significantly reduce dermal toxicity; washing within 1 h may prevent toxicity entirely. M291 skin decontamination kit should be used if available. Superactivated charcoal should be given orally if the toxin is swallowed.

Prophylaxis: The only defense is to prevent exposure by wearing a protective mask and clothing (or topical skin protectant) during an attack. No specific immunotherapy or chemotherapy is available for use in the field.

Isolation and Decontamination: Outer clothing should be removed and exposed skin decontaminated with soap and water. Eye exposure should be treated with copious saline irrigation. Secondary aerosols are not a hazard; however, contact with contaminated skin and clothing can produce secondary dermal exposures. Contact precautions are warranted until decontamination is accomplished. After decontamination, standard precautions are recommended for healthcare workers. A 3%-5% solution of sodium hypochlorite should be used for environmental decontamination.

OVERVIEW

T-2 mycotoxins are trichothecene compounds produced by a variety of filamentous fungi. They are low-molecular-weight compounds that are resistant to heat and UV light making them extremely stable in the environment. Unlike other biological toxins, T-2 mycotoxins are potent dermal irritants and depending on the dose can cause severe skin, and potentially systemic, reactions. Possible dermal, ocular, respiratory, and gastrointestinal exposures should be anticipated after an aerosol attack with mycotoxins.

HISTORY AND SIGNIFICANCE

The potential for T-2 use as a weaponized toxin was suggested during World War II in Orenburg, Russia, where more than 10% of the population was affected when civilians ingested bread unintentionally contaminated with *Fusarium* in wheat flour. Some developed a protracted, ultimately lethal, illness known as "alimentary toxic aleukia" (ATA), characterized initially by abdominal pain, diarrhea, vomiting, prostration, and within days, by fever, chills, myalgias and bone marrow depression with granulocytopenia and secondary sepsis. Survival beyond this point was accompanied by the development of painful pharyngeal / laryngeal ulcerations and diffuse bleeding into the skin (petechiae and ecchymoses), melena, hematochezia, hematuria, hematemesis, epistaxis, and vaginal bleeding. Pancytopenia, and gastrointestinal ulceration and erosion were secondary to the ability of these toxins to profoundly arrest bone marrow and mucosal protein synthesis and cell-cycle progression through DNA replication.

Owing to environmental stability and dissemination potential, T-2 mycotoxins may be weaponized. Controversy still exists over the "yellow rain" incidents where mycotoxins allegedly were released by the Soviet Union and its allies from aircraft during conflicts in Laos (1975-81), Kampuchea (1979-81), and Afghanistan (1979-81). It has been estimated that there were more than 6,300 deaths in Laos, 1,000 in Kampuchea, and 3,042 in Afghanistan. The victims included both unarmed civilians and guerrilla forces. These groups were not protected with gas masks or chemical protective clothing and had little ability to destroy attacking enemy aircraft. The attacks occurred in remote jungle areas, which made definitive confirmation of attacks and recovery of agent extremely difficult. Some have claimed that the "yellow clouds" were, in fact, bee feces produced by swarms of migrating insects. This theory fails to account for the deaths that occurred. Much controversy has centered upon the veracity of eyewitness and victim accounts, but there is evidence for serious consideration of these allegations of biological weapon use. Moreover, Iraq was known to have produced and stockpiled mycotoxins. There was suspicion that T-2 mycotoxins were involved in an Iraqi missile explosion over a US military camp in Saudi Arabia during Operation Desert Storm in 1991.

TOXIN CHARACTERISTICS

The trichothecene mycotoxins are low-molecular-mass (250-500 daltons) nonvolatile compounds produced by filamentous fungi (molds) of the genera *Fusarium, Myrotecium, Trichoderma, Stachybotrys* and others. The structures of approximately 150 trichothecene derivatives have been described. These substances are relatively insoluble in water but are highly soluble in organic solvents such as acetone, ethanol, methanol and propylene glycol. Trichothecenes can vaporize when heated in organic solvents. Extraction of the mycotoxin from fungal cultures yields a yellow-brown liquid that evaporates into a yellow greasy crystalline product (some believe this to be the substance found in "yellow rain"). The trichothecenes are extremely stable and resistant to heat and UV light inactivation. They retain their bioactivity even when autoclaved; heating to 900° F for 10 min or 500°F for 30 min is required for inactivation. A 3-5% solution of sodium hypochlorite is effective for inactivating T-2 mycotoxins and the efficacy can be further enhanced with the addition of small amounts of alkali. U.S. Army decontaminating agents DS-2 and Supertropical bleach inactivate T-2 toxin within 30 to 60 min. In laboratory animals, washing contaminated skin with soap and water within 4 to 6 h removed 80-98% of the toxin, which prevented dermal lesions and death.

MECHANISM OF TOXICITY

Trichothecenes are potent inhibitors of protein synthesis and have a pronounced effect on actively proliferating cells, such as those found in the skin, GI tract, and bone marrow. Because this cytotoxic effect imitates the hematopoietic and lymphoid effects of radiation sickness, the mycotoxins are referred to as "radiomimetic agents." T-2 mycotoxins interfere with peptidyl transferase activity and inhibit either the initiation or elongation of process of translation. The mycotoxins also alter cell membrane structure and function, inhibit mitochondrial respiration, and inactivate certain enzymes.

CLINICAL FEATURES

Clinical signs, symptoms, and severity can vary depending on the route of exposure, toxin concentration, and type of exposure (acute vs. chronic subacute doses). In a biowarfare attack, the toxin(s) can adhere to and penetrate the skin, be inhaled, or be ingested. In the alleged yellow rain incidents, symptoms of exposure from all three routes coexisted. Contaminated clothing may serve as a reservoir for further toxin exposure. Early symptoms beginning within minutes of exposure include burning skin pain, redness, tenderness, blistering, and progression to skin necrosis with leathery blackening and sloughing of large areas of skin. Upper respiratory exposure may result in nasal itching, pain, sneezing, epistaxis, and rhinorrhea. Pulmonary and tracheobronchial toxicity produces dyspnea, wheezing, and cough. Mouth and throat exposure causes pain and blood-tinged saliva and sputum. Anorexia, nausea, vomiting, and watery or bloody diarrhea with cramps and abdominal pain occur with GI toxicity. Eye pain, tearing, redness, foreign body sensation, and blurred vision may follow ocular exposure. Skin symptoms occur in minutes to hours and eye symptoms in minutes. Systemic toxicity can occur via any route of exposure, and results in weakness, prostration, dizziness, ataxia, and loss of coordination. Tachycardia, hypothermia, and hypotension follow in severe cases. Death may occur in minutes, hours, or days. The most common symptoms are vomiting, diarrhea, skin involvement with burning pain, redness and pruritus, rash or blisters, bleeding, and dyspnea. A late effect of systemic absorption is pancytopenia, predisposing to bleeding and sepsis.

DIAGNOSIS

Clinical and epidemiological findings provide clues to the diagnosis. High attack rates, dead animals of multiple species, along with physical evidence such as yellow, red, green, or other pigmented oily liquids, suggest mycotoxin exposure. Rapid onset of symptoms in minutes to hours supports a diagnosis of a chemical or toxin attack. In addition, the coexistence of cutaneous, ocular, respiratory, and GI symptoms may support the suspicion of mycotoxin exposure. Mustard and other vesicant agents must be considered, especially there is a distinctive odor, visible residue is present, and along with a rapid detection by a field chemical test (M8 paper, M256 kit). Symptoms from mustard toxicity are also delayed for several hours after exposure. Inhalation of SEB or ricin aerosols can cause fever, cough, dyspnea, and wheezing but does not involve the skin.

There are several commercial immunoassay kits on the market that detect trichothecene mycotoxins in grain and feed; however, a rapid diagnostic test is unavailable for field clinical use. Serum and urine should be collected and sent to a reference laboratory for antigen detection. The mycotoxins and metabolites are eliminated in the urine and feces; 50-75% is eliminated within 24 h; however, metabolites can be detected as late as 28 days after exposure. Pathologic specimens may include blood, urine, lung, liver, and stomach contents. Environmental and clinical samples can be tested using a gas liquid chromatography (GLC) or high-performance liquid chromatography (HPLC)-mass spectrometry (MS) combination technique. GLC-MS and HPLC-MS are the best and most sensitive methods for detecting mycotoxins. This system can detect as little as 0.1-1.0 parts per billion of T-2, which is sensitive enough to measure T-2 levels in the plasma of toxin victims.

MEDICAL MANAGEMENT

No specific antidote or therapeutic regimen is currently available. All therapy is supportive. If a soldier is unprotected during an attack, the outer uniform should be removed as soon as possible. The skin should be thoroughly washed with soap and water. This may reduce dermal toxicity, even if delayed 4-6 h after exposure. The M291 skin decontamination kit can also be used to remove skin-adherent T-2. XE-556 resin, which is similar to the XE-555 resin in the M291 kit, was shown to be effective in the physical removal of T-2 toxin from the skin in animal studies. Treatment for cutaneous involvement resembles standard burn care. Standard therapy for poison ingestion, including the use of superactivated charcoal to absorb swallowed T-2 toxin, should be administered to victims of an unprotected aerosol attack. Respiratory support may be necessary. The eyes should be irrigated with normal saline or water to remove toxin. Contaminated clothing as well as wash waste from the decontamination process should be exposed to bleach (5% sodium hypochlorite) for 6 h or more to neutralize any residual myxotoxins. Some survival benefit was seen with administration of dexamethasone, diphenhydramine, naloxone, methylthiazolidine-4-carboxylate, metoclopramide, magenesium sulfate, and sodium bicarbonate in animal studies. No similar studies have been conducted in humans.

PROPHYLAXIS

Physical protection of the skin, mucous membranes, and airway (use of chemical protective mask and clothing) are the only proven effective methods of protection during an attack. Skin exposure reduction paste against chemical warfare agents (SERPACWA) has been shown to block dermal irritation in animal studies and can be applied at closure points of chemical over-garments as well as any skin-exposed areas. Immunologic (vaccines and monoclonal antibodies) and chemoprotective pretreatments are being studied in animal models, but are not available for field use. Soap and water washing, even 1 h after dermal exposure to T-2, effectively prevents dermal toxicity.

EMERGING THREATS AND POTENTIAL BIOLOGICAL WEAPONS

OVERVIEW

The evolving biowarfare threat is becoming more complex because of increased agent variety, sophistication, and the feasibility of *in vitro* genetic modification. Although anthrax will remain an attractive option for many state and non-state perpetrators, some groups may focus on new types of viral and bacterial agents. The availability of biowarfare -relevant technology, materials, information, and expertise has increased, as has publicity about potential vulnerabilities. Novel genetic engineering and other advances in biotechnology provide powerful capabilities to modify virtually any bio-agent, affecting characteristics such as enhanced agent virulence, increased environmental stability, resistance to medical countermeasures, and defeat of physical barriers and bio-detectors.

While there are no simple solutions to the threat of emerging infectious disease and novel biological weapons, expansion of U.S. national expertise and fostering of new international partnerships may greatly help create synergies for the detection and deterrence of biological threats. The type of situational awareness needed for a global pandemic overlaps with that needed to detect a major bioterrorist campaign.

Finally, along with the wider civilian community, DoD has recognized that emerging infectious diseases represent an uncontrolled source of mayhem, which could be harnessed for nefarious purposes. The appearance of a new or reemerging infectious disease can have global implications. During the past 20 yrs, over 30 novel lethal pathogens have been identified. In addition to the traditional bioagents such as anthrax and plague, more familiar reemerging pathogens, such as influenza, represent significant future threats to both military and civilian populations. This is especially true since modern molecular biology techniques allow modified or completely new organisms to be made in the laboratory.

The 2010 Quadrennial Defense Review placed increased emphasis on non-proliferation and emerging threats and recognized the challenge of developing countermeasures against non-traditional agents. Addressing these novel bio-agents is a central objective of the Homeland Security Presidential Directive/HSPD-18, *Medical Countermeasures against Weapons of*

Mass Destruction (January 31, 2007), coordinated with the Executive Office of the President, DoD, and Department of Health and Human Services (DHHS). As technological advances continue to evolve, our defensive capabilities should preferably include a two-tiered approach for development and acquisition of medical countermeasures, which will balance the immediate need to provide a capability to mitigate the most catastrophic of the current CBRN threats, with long-term requirements to develop more flexible, broader spectrum countermeasures to address future threats.

HSPD-18 frames the biological threat spectrum into four distinct categories, the last three of which concern non-traditional agents.

(a) Traditional agents: naturally occurring microorganisms or toxins with the potential to be disseminated to cause mass casualties (e.g., *Bacillus anthracis* (anthrax) and *Yersinia pestis* (plague)).

(b) Enhanced agents: traditional agents that have been modified or selected to enhance their ability to harm human populations or circumvent current countermeasures, such as a bacterium that has been modified to resist antibiotic treatment.

(c) Emerging agents: previously unrecognized pathogens that might be naturally occurring and present a serious risk to human populations (e.g., severe acute respiratory syndrome (SARS) virus).

(d) Advanced agents: novel pathogens or biologicals that have been artificially engineered in the laboratory to bypass traditional medical countermeasures or produce a more severe or otherwise enhanced spectrum of disease.

DOD CHEMICAL AND BIOLOGICAL DEFENSE PROGRAM (CBDP)

Enacted by Congress in 1993, Public Law 103-160 created the DoD Chemical and Biological Defense Program (CBDP). The Assistant to the Secretary of Defense for Nuclear and Chemical and Biological Defense Programs [ATSD(NCB)] is the principal advisor to the Secretary and Deputy Secretary of Defense, and the Under Secretary of Defense for Acquisition, Technology, and Logistics (USD(AT&L)) on nuclear energy, nuclear weapons, and chemical and biological defense and provides overall coordination, integration, and oversight of the CBDP.

Novel bio-agents and emerging infectious diseases present complex challenges for the nation and our warfighters. The CBDP is implementing steps to assess and mitigate risks associated with these emerging threats, including analysis of non-traditional agents and the expansion of the Transformational Medical Technologies (TMT) Initiative.

Transformational Medical Technologies: The DOD's TMT mission is to protect the warfighter from emerging and genetically engineered biological threats by providing a robust response capability ranging from identification of pathogens through to the development of medical countermeasures. TMT is pursuing technologies to characterize unknown pathogens and rapidly develop medical countermeasures to newly identified threats. The program intends to spur innovative research to develop broad-spectrum medical countermeasures that are peer-reviewed and FDA approved.

The TMT initiative is a vital part of the National Biodefense Strategy and the Integrated National Biodefense Medical Countermeasures Portfolio (INBDP), which is coordinated with the Executive Office of the President, DoD, and DHHS. This active interagency participation is essential to the development and implementation of an effective biodefense capability for the nation. The overarching goal of the TMT is to provide proof-of-process for development of platform technologies that allow for the rapid development of Medical Countermeasures (MCMs); determination of the genetic sequences for pertinent threats against which to screen, identify, and characterize potential biodefense threats; and development of needed broad-spectrum countermeasures for viral and intracellular bacterial (ICB) pathogens.

The TMT Initiative commenced in the third quarter of FY 2006 and integrates the science and technology capabilities of the Defense Threat Reduction Agency (DTRA) with the acquisition capabilities of the DoD Joint Program Executive Office for Chemical and Biological Defense (JPEO-CBD) into a single process responsible for the end-to-end development and delivery of capabilities enabling rapid response to genetically engineered and emerging biological threats. The TMT initiative receives program oversight from the ATSD(NCB) and guidance from an executive office made up of senior leadership from both the JPEO-CBD and DTRA.

Defense Advanced Research Projects Agency (DARPA): The CBDP has a memorandum of understanding with DARPA to manage the Advanced Manufacturing of Pharmaceuticals (AMP) program. The goal of this program is to create a rapid, flexible, and cost-effective production technology capable of producing millions of doses of protein for a new therapeutic monoclonal antibody or vaccine within 12 wks of notification at low cost and with an unprecedented purity for any emerging infectious threat.

A second DARPA initiative to respond faster to unknown or emerging novel biothreat agents is their 7-day Biodefense Initiative. Under this effort, countermeasures could be developed for multiple unrelated infectious agents within 7 days. This two-phase program focused on preventing infection, sustaining survival until a curative response is available, providing transient immunity, and speeding the onset of adaptive immunity. The goal is to develop highly innovative approaches to counter any known, unknown, naturally occurring or engineered pathogen. Particular interest focuses on new approaches that obviate traditional and rate-limiting steps (e.g., pathogen isolation, culture, identification, antigen processing by the immune system, and onset of adaptive immunity).

BIOLOGICAL THREAT REDUCTION PROGRAM (BTRP)

Sen. Richard Lugar and former Sen. Sam Nunn produced the Nunn-Lugar Act in 1991, establishing the Cooperative Threat Reduction (CTR) Program. The CTR program helps states of the former Soviet Union to safeguard and dismantle their enormous stockpiles of nuclear, chemical and biological weapons, related materials, and delivery systems. DTRA executes the CTR program and works in coordination with partner governments and other U.S. government agencies who administer related projects.

While the initial focus of the CTR program has been on the most pressing nuclear proliferation threats, funding was also directed toward improving the physical protection, safety and security of facilities that housed dangerous bio-agents under the cooperative Biological Threat Reduction program (BTRP). The BTRP helps build capacity in partner countries by improving detection, diagnostics, monitoring, and reporting of endemic and epidemic diseases whether naturally occurring or man-made.

The BTRP is developing cooperative disease surveillance programs with partner nation governments and helping partners comply with the World Health Assembly (WHA) International Health Regulations (IHR) and reporting guidelines for the World Organization for Animal Health (OIE) and the United Nation's Food and Agricultural Organization (FAO).

In 2009, the National Academy of Sciences (NAS) congressionally-mandated report, "*Global Security Engagement: A New Model for Cooperative*

Threat Reduction", recommended an expanded Nunn-Lugar model of global security engagement to counter the 21st century terrorist threats. The Nunn Lugar Global Cooperation Initiative gives higher priority to global engagement and surveillance for biological threats.

Another primary mission of the BTRP is to help consolidate Especially Dangerous Pathogen (EDP) collections, including those on the U.S. Select Agent List, into one or two safe, secure facilities per country and work to prevent the sale, theft, diversion, or accidental release of biological weapons related materials, technology, and expertise.

While BTRP's activities since 1991 have been focused on former Soviet countries (Armenia, Azerbaijan, Georgia, Kazakhstan, Ukraine, Uzbekistan), there is now the organizational mandate for similar work in Afghanistan, Pakistan, and Sub-Saharan Africa under the rubric of the Cooperative Biological Engagement Program (CBEP).

EMERGING INFECTIOUS DISEASES

Emerging infectious diseases are those that are: (1) newly recognized as occurring in humans (or animals or plants), (2) newly occurring in a different population than previously, (3) affecting greater numbers of individuals, or, (4) has evolving new attributes (e.g., resistance or virulence). Even though some "emerging" diseases have been recognized for more than 20 yrs (e.g., AIDS, Lyme disease, Legionnaire's disease), their importance has not diminished and the factors associated with their emergence are still relevant.

Many factors contribute to the emergence of new diseases, notably: environmental changes; increased global travel and trade; social upheaval; and genetic changes in infectious agents, host, or vector populations. Once a new disease is introduced into a susceptible human population, it may spread rapidly and could challenge the medical and public health infrastructures. If the disease is severe, it may lead to social disruption and cause severe economic impact. Novel infectious agents such as SARS or the 2009 H1N1 influenza virus appear to be occurring with increasing frequency and with a greater potential for serious consequences.

In a 2008 study funded by the National Science Foundation (NSF), about two-thirds of emerging infections were found to be zoonotic (animal in origin) and the majority of those came from wild animals (e.g., SARS, Ebola virus). Important geographic areas of emergence include Sub-Saharan Africa, India and China, and Europe, and North and South America. New pathogens may be transmitted directly by hunting or accidental contact, while others are transferred from wildlife to livestock to people (e.g., Malaysia's Nipah virus). Humans have evolved little resistance to zoonotic diseases, so the diseases can be extraordinarily lethal.

About 20% of known emerging infections are caused by multidrug-resistant strains of previously known pathogens, including tuberculosis. Wealthier nations' increasing dependence on, and misuse of, antibiotics augments the proliferation of such dangerous variants of common bacteria. An example is enterotoxigenic *Escherichia coli*, now spread widely with great speed because products like raw vegetables are processed in huge, centralized facilities, and hastily packaged for rapid onward shipment and consumption.

President Barack Obama announced, in his 2010 State of the Union Address, that "We are launching new initiatives that will give us the capacity to respond faster and more effectively to bioterrorism or an infectious disease".

The U.S. National Security Strategy (NSS), released in May 2010, provides a mandate to reduce the risk associated with unintentional or deliberate outbreaks of infectious disease, pursue new strategies to protect against biological attacks, and promote global health security generally.

The CBDP formally added emerging infectious diseases to the biodefense mission set in October 2009. Subsequently, DoD executed chemical and biodefense program funds for emerging infectious disease preparedness and response activities. The CBDP Fiscal Year 2012-2017 Program Strategy Guidance declared that "infectious diseases, either emerging or reemerging, must be a focus of DoD, and we must be ready to play an important role in responding to pandemics, whether naturally occurring (H1N1) or not (smallpox)."

The key to recognizing new or emerging infectious diseases, and to tracking the prevalence of more established ones, is surveillance. Biosurveillance is the prerequisite to effectively addressing the array of biological threats to our national security from natural, accidental, and intentional origins.

Emergence of pandemic influenza, Ebola virus, Marburg, SARS, anthrax, West Nile virus, prion diseases, multidrug-resistant tuberculosis (MDR-TB), and scores of other "new" diseases remind clinicians and public health officials to remain vigilant for outbreaks of novel or unexplained diseases. These emerging infections have a potential to become future biological threats. Natural emerging disease outbreaks may be difficult to distinguish from the intentional introduction of infectious diseases for nefarious purposes; hence, consideration must be given to this possibility before any question of etiology is considered settled.

Because emerging diseases are so diverse, exotic, and various according to different geographic locations, their complete description is beyond the scope of this handbook. Summaries of a few recent emerging infections follow but one should be mindful that the most worrisome pathogen may well be the one not yet recognized.

Pandemic Influenza: The threat for pandemic spread of human influenza is substantial. The pathogenicity of influenza viruses is directly related to their ability to rapidly alter their eight viral RNA segments. New antigenic variation results in the formation of new hemagglutinin (HA) or neuraminidase (NA) surface glycoproteins, which may go unrecognized by an immune system primed against heterologous strains.

Two distinct phenomena contribute to a renewed susceptibility to influenza infection among persons previously infected. Clinically significant variants of influenza A viruses may result from mutations in the HA and NA genes, expressed as minor structural changes in the viral surface proteins. As few as four amino acid substitutions in any two antigenic sites can cause a clinically significant variation. These minor changes result in an altered virus able to circumvent host immunity. Additionally, genetic reassortment between avian and human, or avian and porcine, influenza viruses may lead to major changes in HA or NA surface proteins known as "antigenic shift." In contrast to the gradual evolution of strains subject to "antigenic drift", antigenic shift occurs when an influenza virus with a completely novel HA or NA formation moves into humans from other host species. Global pandemics such as in 2009 have resulted from such antigenic shifts.

Influenza causes more than 30,000 deaths and more than 100,000 hospitalizations annually in the U.S. Pandemic influenza viruses have emerged regularly in 10- to 50-yr cycles for the last several centuries. During the last century, influenza pandemics occurred four times: 1918 ("Spanish influenza", a H1N1 virus), 1957 (Asian influenza, an H2N2 subtype strain), in 1968 (Hong Kong influenza, an H3N2 variant), and most recently, in 2009 (California H1N1 influenza).

The 1918 influenza pandemic illustrates a worst-case public health scenario: it caused 675,000 deaths in the U.S. and 20-40 million deaths worldwide. Morbidity in most communities was between 25-40%, and case fatality rate averaged 2.5%. A re-emergent 1918-like influenza virus would have tremendous societal effects, even in the event that antiviral medications proved effective.

The 1957-58 pandemic caused 66,000 excess deaths, and the 1968 pandemic caused 34,000 excess deaths in the United States.

In April 2009, an outbreak of influenza-like illness occurred in Mexico and the U.S.; the CDC reported seven cases of a novel A/H1N1 influenza virus. The disease then spread very rapidly, with the number of confirmed cases rising to 2,099 by May 7, 2009, despite aggressive measures taken by the Mexican government to curb the spread of the disease. On June 11, 2009, the WHO declared an H1N1 pandemic (pandemic alert phase 6), the first global influenza pandemic since the 1968 Hong Kong flu. Fortunately, the 2009 H1N1 virus was fatal in 0.01–0.03% of those infected, making it considerably less lethal than previous pandemic strains (1918 H1N1 virus was 100 times more lethal). However, incidence and case fatality rates (CFRs) for the 2009 H1N1 pandemic varied by age. Children (age 5-14 yrs) had the highest estimated incidence rate and the lowest CFR (0.01% CFR), whereas elders (age, ≥65) had the lowest estimated incidence rate and highest CFR (0.98% CFR).

The emergence of the pandemic 2009 influenza virus reaffirmed the world's susceptibility to reemerging infections. The 1918 virus was thought to have emerged from birds almost simultaneously into humans and swine. In contrast to the 1918 virus, the 2009 influenza virus contained genes from five different flu viruses: North American swine influenza, North American avian influenza, human influenza and two swine influenza viruses typically found in Asia and Europe.

Wild aquatic birds are the reservoirs of all subtypes of influenza A virus, where they generally cause no harm. Transmission from aquatic birds to humans was originally hypothesized to require infection of an intermediate, such as a pig, that has both human-specific and avian-specific receptors on its respiratory epithelium. Scientists understand that influenza A viruses can transmit directly from birds to humans.

But pigs remain a natural "mixing vessel" for influenza viruses because they can be infected both by avian and human influenza viruses allowing for the reassortment between avian and human influenza viruses to occur. When pigs become simultaneously infected with more than one virus, the viruses can swap genes, producing new variants which can pass to humans and sometimes spread among them. In June 2010, scientists from Hong Kong reported reassortment of the 2009 pandemic virus with viruses previously found in pigs, forming a new hybrid swine flu virus.

Avian Influenza: "Avian influenza virus" usually refers to influenza A viruses primarily found in birds. However, occasional confirmed cases of human infection with several subtypes of avian influenza virus have been reported since 1997. Most human cases of avian influenza infection have resulted from direct contact with infected poultry (e.g., domestic chickens, ducks, and turkeys) or surfaces contaminated with secretion/

excretions from infected birds. The spread of avian influenza viruses from an ill person to another person has been reported very rarely, and transmission has been limited, inefficient and unsustained.

An epizootic of highly pathogenic avian influenza virus (HPAI H5N1) emerged in Southeast Asia in 2003 before spreading to other continents, mostly in animals (poultry, aquatic birds), but also in humans. By January 2011, over 6,780 animal outbreaks of HPAI H5N1 had been reported in 51 countries. Several countries (e.g., Egypt, Indonesia) suspended animal surveillance for HPAI H5N1 several years earlier even though they had accounted for 20% of the world's animal outbreaks. As of June 2011, 562 cases of human HPAI H5N1 and 329 deaths had been reported in 15 countries.

Avian influenza in humans presents like other types of influenza : usually beginning with fever, chills, headaches and myalgias, and often involving the upper and lower respiratory tract with development of cough, dyspnea, and, in severe cases, acute respiratory distress syndrome (ARDS). Laboratory findings may include pancytopenia, lymphopenia, elevated liver enzymes, hypoxia, positive RT-PCR for H5N1 and positive neutralization assay for H5N1.

Because all influenza viruses have a tendency to genetically alter and because the HPAI H5N1 is known to cause human infections, scientists remain concerned that HPAI H5N1 viruses have the potential to change into forms capable of spreading readily from person to person. If HPAI H5N1 were to gain the capacity to do so, another influenza pandemic could begin. Experts from around the world continue to monitor for potential changes in HPAI H5N1 and changes in patterns of human infection and work to prevent a new pandemic.

SARS and SARS-CoV: Another example of zoonotic spread of a new disease was the emergence of severe acute respiratory syndrome (SARS) in Southeast Asia in 2003 due to a novel *Coronavirus* which jumped the species barrier from animals to humans and rapidly spread to 29 countries in less than 90 days. As of today, the spread of SARS has been fully contained, with the last infected human case seen in June 2003 (disregarding a laboratory exposure in 2004).

Before a case definition had been clearly established, Chinese authorities reported to the WHO over 300 cases of an atypical pneumonia with five related deaths; all originated from Guangdong Province in China during

February 2003. The infection quickly spread by air travel to Hong Kong, and from there to Vietnam, Canada, and other locations. Only eight laboratory-confirmed cases occurred in the U.S. but there is concern that the U.S. population is vulnerable to a widespread outbreak such as occurred in 2003.

SARS was still considered a relatively rare disease with a total of 8,273 cases reported as of July 2003 with 775 deaths for a CFR 9.4%. In late May 2003, studies from samples of wild animals sold as food in the local market in Guangdong, China found that the SARS *Coronavirus* could be isolated from palm civets (*Paguma* sp.), but the animals did not always show clinical signs. The preliminary conclusion was that the SARS virus crossed from palm civets to humans, and more than 10,000 masked palm civets were destroyed in Guangdong Province. In 2005, phylogenetic analysis of these viruses indicated a high probability that SARS *Coronavirus* originated in bats and spread to humans either directly, or through animals held in Chinese markets. The bats did not show any visible signs of disease, but are the likely natural reservoirs of SARS-like coronaviruses (SARS-CoV).

BIOENGINEERED THREATS

As scientists develop more sophisticated laboratory procedures and increase their understanding of molecular biology and the human genetic code, the possibility of bioengineering virulent, antibiotic-resistant and vaccine-resistant pathogens for nefarious uses will increase. It is theoretically possible to synthesize and weaponize certain biological response modifiers (BMRs), as well as to engineer genomic weapons capable of inserting novel DNA into host cells. The potential to cause widespread disease and death is incalculable. Fortunately, scientists and policy makers have begun to address the issue and a robust research agenda to develop medical countermeasures is underway.

Genetic vectors: Genetic vectors are used to transfer human and foreign genes into human cells for therapeutic purposes. Viral vectors, such as adenovirus, vaccinia, and other associated viruses, as well as naked or plasmid DNA, have been engineered for the sole purpose of delivering foreign genes into new cells.

These highly specialized genetic vectors are used in gene therapy research and are genetically modified through the deletion of several important viral genes. This creates space for foreign genes and renders the virus incapable of replication once inserted into the host genome.

For the moment, adenovirus and adeno-associated vectors seem to be the favorite viral vectors for experiments involving the introduction of foreign genes into human cell types. These vectors have high transduction efficiency, ability to invade non-dividing cells, and the ability to infect a wide variety of cell-types. Most successful gene therapy experiments have involved the use of these viral vectors as the vehicle for the introduction of new genes. This technology offers the promise of treating or curing a myriad of human ailments but also offers the potential for misuse.

Genomic manipulation: Genomic manipulation to engineer new bioterror weapons has been a concern long before the Human Genome Project was completed in 2003. However, it is now possible to synthesize a potential pathogen only using its DNA sequence, without access to actual cultures or stock of the agent. Complete or partial genomic sequence data for many of the most lethal human pathogens (such as anthrax and plague bacilli and the smallpox virus) are published and widely available through internet sites, often with free unrestricted access.

Biosecurity initiatives have emerged over the past decade designed to regulate the laboratory use and access to pathogens. However, because of the growth in DNA synthesis technology, solely restricting access to such pathogens will not provide total security. Technology to synthesize organisms genetically becomes more readily available every year.

The rapid advance of biotechnology has tremendous potential to alter the present and future threat of biological weapons. In addition to this enormous explosion in our knowledge of human pathogens is a parallel understanding of the complexities of the human immune response to foreign agents and toxins. With this increase in scientific knowledge has come the power to manipulate the immune system at its most fundamental level. As we prepare for future threats, we must not ignore the potential quantum leap biotechnology offers our potential enemies in developing new biowarfare threats. There is evidence that novel bio-agents have already been produced by former adversaries. Examples of such novel threat agents and the potential effects they might have on human subjects have been detailed in the scientific and popular literature. Examples of novel biologic threats that could be produced through the use of genetic engineering technology include:

- Microorganisms resistant to antibiotics, standard vaccines and/or therapeutics

- Innocuous microorganisms genetically altered to produce a toxin, poisonous substance, or endogenous bioregulator
- Microorganisms possessing enhanced aerosol and environmental stability characteristics
- Immunologically altered microorganisms which are able to defeat standard threat identification, and/or diagnostic methods
- Combinations of the above with improved delivery systems

The concept of "genomic warfare" is highly speculative and beyond the scope of this handbook. Undoubtedly as scientific understanding of this technology increases and becomes more widely available, the threat of the development and use of genomic weapons will increase as will the challenge to develop effective medical countermeasures.

Ultimately, the capacity to create deadly new organisms through genetic engineering is restrained in large part by technical knowledge and opportunity. What may appear straightforward for skilled scientists can be impossibly difficult for the untrained and unequipped. However, a determined person with the appropriate knowledge, skills, or access to personnel with such skills may succeed in malevolent creation of genetically engineered microorganisms.

Bioregulators (or modulators): Bioregulators or modulators are biochemical compounds, such as peptides, that occur naturally in organisms. Advances in biotechnology have created the potential for the misuse of bioregulators as biological weapons. As bioweapons, they could damage the nervous system, alter moods, trigger psychological changes and kill. The potential military or terrorist use of bioregulators is somewhat similar to that of toxins.

Many bioregulators can be used to cause illness, but only a few can threaten civilian populations on a large scale. If released upon a civilian population in sufficient quantity and concentration, they could pose significant challenges for public health and medical responses.

Biological Response Modifiers (BRMs): Biological response modifiers (BRMs) direct the myriad complex interactions of the human immune system. BRMs include erythropoietins, interferons, interleukins, colony-stimulating factors, stem cell growth factors, monoclonal antibodies, tumor necrosis factor inhibitors, and vaccines.

A growing understanding of the structure and function of various BRMs has resulted in many novel compounds including synthetic analgesics, antioxidants, antiviral, and antibacterial substances. For example, BRMs are used to treat debilitating rheumatoid arthritis by targeting cytokines that contribute to the disease process, to reduce symptoms and decrease inflammation. Recently marketed BRM-based medications include etanercept (*Enbrel*) and infliximab (*Remicade*), both of which have been used to target the tumor necrosis factor alpha (TNFα) cytokine, as well as anakinra (*Kineret*), which targets interleuken –1 (IL-1).

More of these new drugs are currently in development. It can be easily imagined that research to develop various BRMs could be subverted to a malicious end. That is, instead of using BRMs to suppress cancer growth or disease susceptibility, such compounds could potentially be developed to have the opposite effect, causing illness and death to those exposed.

PERSONAL PROTECTION

The currently fielded chemical protective equipment which includes the protective mask, the Joint Services lightweight integrated suit technology (JSLIST) chemical protective overgarment (CPO), which replaces the battle dress overgarment (BDO); protective gloves; protective footwear covers, and multipurpose rain/snow/CW overboots (MULO) will effectively protect against a bio-agent attack.

The standard issue mask, the M40, is available in three sizes, and when worn correctly, will protect the face, eyes, and respiratory tract. The M40 employs a single, standard screw-on C2A1 filter element which incorporates two separate but complementary mechanisms: 1) impaction and adsorption of agent molecules onto ASC Whetlerite carbon filtration medium, and 2) static electrical attraction of particles which are able to pass carbon filtration medium on first pass. Proper maintenance and periodic replacement of the crucial filter elements is of utmost importance. The filter MUST be replaced when:

- The elements become immersed in water, crushed, cut, or otherwise damaged.
- Excessive breathing resistance is encountered.
- The "ALL CLEAR" signal is given after exposure to a bio-agent.
- Thirty days have elapsed in the combat theater of operations (the filters must be replaced every 30 days once opened).
- Supply bulletins indicate lot number expiration.
- So ordered by the unit commander.

The filter element must only be changed in an un-contaminated environment. Two styles of optical inserts for the protective mask are available for personnel requiring visual correction. The wire frame style is considered to be the safer of the two and is more easily fitted into the mask. A prong-type optical insert is also available. A drinking tube on the mask can be used while in a contaminated environment. Note that the wearer should disinfect the canteen and tube by wiping with a 5% hypochlorite solution before use.

The Joint Service General Protective Mask (JSGPM, US Army XM-50) is a lightweight protective mask incorporating state-of-the-art technology. It is composed of heavy rubber, has a chlorobutyl/silicone base with a polynomial spline eye lens, incorporates a hydration port, and has a 50% performance improvement over the M40, for Joint force protection requirements. It provides above-the-neck, head-eye-respiratory protection against CBRN threats, including toxic industrial chemicals. JSGPM will replace the M40/M42 series of protective masks for the Army and Marines, and the MCU-2/P series of protective masks for the Air Force and Navy. It is intended to interface with Joint service vehicles, weapons, communication systems, individual clothing and protective equipment, and CBRN personal protective equipment. JSGPM production and fielding began in 2008, and will continue until the Service's requirements are filled.

The JSLIST is available 7 sizes, woodland and desert patterns, and can be used for 45 days in an uncontaminated environment. Once opened it can be laundered up to six times and may be worn for 24 continuous h in a contaminated environment. The JSLIST is replaced by using the MOPP-gear exchange procedure described in the *Soldier's Manual of Common Tasks*. The discarded suit should be incinerated or buried. Chemical protective gloves and overboots come in various sizes and are both made from butyl rubber. They may be decontaminated and reissued. The gloves and overboots must be visually inspected and decontaminated as needed after every 12 h of exposure in a contaminated environment. While the protective equipment will protect against bio-agents, it is noteworthy that even standard uniform clothing of good quality affords a reasonable protection against dermal exposure of surfaces covered.

The BDO is a two-layer, two piece garment consisting of coat and trousers. A water-repellant treated nylon/cotton twill outer layer, with an inner layer of polyurethane foam/nylon tricot laminate impregnated with activated charcoal. Available in 8 sizes, the BDO is no longer in production, and is being replaced by the JSLIST.

Those casualties unable to continue wearing protective equipment should be held and / or transported within patient protective wraps designed to protect the patient against further chemical-biological agent exposure. These wraps consist of a charcoal lining similar to the BDO, with a bottom layer of impermeable rubber. Healthcare personnel transporting such patients may want to consider adding a filter blower unit to generate overpressure, and thereby enhance protection and provide cooling.

Collective protection by using either a hardened or unhardened shelter equipped with an air filtration unit providing overpressure can protect personnel in a biologically contaminated environment. An airlock ensures that no contamination will be brought into the shelter. In the absence of a dedicated structure, enhanced protection can be afforded within most buildings by sealing cracks and entry ports, and providing air filtration with high efficiency particulate air (HEPA) filters within existing ventilation systems. The key problem is that availability of these shelters can be limited in military situations, costly to produce and maintain, and difficult to deploy. Personnel must be decontaminated before entering the collective protection unit.

The inhalational route is the most important route of exposure to bio-agents. Bio-agents can be dispersed as aerosols from point or line source disseminations. Unlike some chemical threats, aerosols of bio-agents disseminated by line source munitions (e.g., sprayed by low-flying aircraft or speedboats along the coast) do not leave hazardous environmental residue (although anthrax spores may persist and could pose a hazard near the dissemination line). In contrast, aerosols generated by point-source munitions (i.e., stationary aerosol generator, bomblets, etc.) are more apt to produce ground contamination, but only in the immediate vicinity of dissemination. Point-source munitions leave an obvious signature that may alert the field commander that a BW attack has occurred. Because point-source munitions always leave an agent residue, this evidence can be useful for detection and identification purposes.

Aerosol delivery systems for bioagents most commonly generate invisible clouds with particles or droplets of < 10 μmm. They can remain suspended for extensive periods. The major risk in such an attack is pulmonary retention of inhaled particles. To a much lesser extent, some particles may adhere to an individual or his clothing, especially near the face. The effective area covered varies with many factors, including wind speed, humidity, and sunlight. In the absence of an effective real-time detection and alarm systems or direct observation of an attack, the first clue may be mass casualties fitting a clinical pattern compatible with one of the bio-agents. This may occur hours, days, or weeks after an attack.

Toxins may cause direct pulmonary effects or be absorbed and cause systemic toxicity. They are frequently more potent by inhalation than by any other route. A unique clinical feature may be seen which is not observed by other routes (e.g., pulmonary edema after SEB exposure). Mucous membranes, including conjunctivae, are also vulnerable to many bio-agents. Physical protection is then quite important and the use of full-face masks equipped with small-particle filters, like the chemical protective masks, assumes a high degree of importance.

With reference to force protection, other routes for delivering bio-agents are thought to be less significant than inhalation, but are nonetheless potentially significant. Contamination of food and water supplies, either deliberately or incidentally after an aerosol attack, represents a hazard for infection or intoxication by ingestion. Determination as to whether food and water supplies are free from contamination is always important, and should be made by appropriate preventive medicine authorities in the event of a bioattack.

Intact skin provides an excellent barrier against most bio-agents -- T-2 mycotoxins are the sole exception, due to their dermal activity. It is also important to consider that, mucous membranes and abrasions, or otherwise damaged integument, can allow for passage of some bioagents, and should therefore be protected in the event of an attack.

DECONTAMINATION

Biological contamination is the introduction of infectious agents to a body surface, food or water, or other inanimate object. In this context, decontamination involves either disinfection or sterilization to reduce microorganisms to a safe level on contaminated articles, thus rendering them suitable for use. Disinfection is the selective reduction of undesirable microbes to a level below that required for transmission. Sterilization is the killing of all organisms.

Decontamination methods have always played an important role in the control of infectious diseases. However, the most effective means of rendering microbes harmless (e.g., toxic chemical sterilization) may be impractical, as these methods may injure people, or damage equipment. Bio-agents may be also be decontaminated by mechanical, chemical or physical methods.

1) Mechanical decontamination involves measures to remove but not necessarily neutralize an agent. An example is drinking water filtration to remove certain water-borne pathogens (e.g., *Dracunculus medinensis, Naegleria fowleri*), or the use of an air filter to remove aerosolized anthrax spores, or soap and water to wash agent from the skin.

2) Chemical decontamination renders bio-agents harmless by the use of disinfectants that may be a liquid, gas, or aerosol. Factors impacting effectiveness include contact time, solution concentration, composition of the contaminated surface, and characteristics of the agent to be decontaminated. Some disinfectants are harmful to humans, animals, the environment, and/or materiel.

3) Physical processes (heat, radiation) are other methods that can be employed for decontaminating objects.

It is important that, given the characteristic incubation periods of bio-agents, significant time may have elapsed between the attack and the patients' presentation with illness due to the attack. During this time it is quite probable that external decontamination of any residual agent may have already occurred through natural means. Thus, it is only in rare circumstances that patients presenting with illness due to a biological attack will require purposeful external decontamination.

Dermal exposure to a suspected biological aerosol should be immediately and vigorously treated by soap and water washing. This removes nearly all the agent from the skin surface. Hypochlorite solution or other disinfectants are reserved for gross contamination (i.e., after the spill of solid or liquid agent from munitions directly onto the skin). In the absence of chemical agent or gross biological contamination, these disinfectants will confer no additional benefit, may be caustic, and may predispose patients to colonization and resistant superinfection by eliminating the normal skin flora. Grossly contaminated skin surfaces should be washed with a 0.5% sodium hypochlorite solution, if available, with a contact time of 10 to 15 min. If reaerosolization of agent is a concern due to the presence of gross contaminant, a damp cloth or towel should be placed directly over the area and a 5% solution of hypochlorite (or equivalent disinfectant) should be liberally applied to saturate the gross contaminant. The saturated fabric/bio-agent should then be properly disposed of per established protocol.

Ampules of calcium hypochlorite (HTH) are currently fielded in the Chemical Agent Decon Set for mixing hypochlorite solutions. The 0.5% solution can be made by adding one 6-ounce container of calcium hypochlorite to 5 gallons of water. The 5% solution can be made by adding eight 6-ounce ampules of calcium hypochlorite to 5 gallons of water. These solutions evaporate quickly at high temperatures. If made in advance, they should be stored in closed containers. Chlorine solutions should always be placed in distinctly marked containers, as without markings it is very difficult to tell the difference between the 5% chlorine solution and the 0.5% solution.

A 0.5% sodium hypochlorite solution is made of one part Clorox and nine parts water (1:9) as standard stock Clorox is a 5.25% sodium hypochlorite solution. The solution is then applied with a cloth or swab. The solution should be made fresh daily with the pH in the alkaline range.

Generally, soap and water wash is the preferred method for bio-agent decontamination of patients. Chlorine solution must NOT be used in (1) open body-cavity wounds (as it may lead to the formation of adhesions), or (2) brain and spinal cord injuries. However, this solution (0.5% strength) may be instilled into non-cavity wounds and then removed by suction to an appropriate disposal container. Within about 5 m, this contaminated solution will be neutralized and non-hazardous. Copious irrigation with saline or other surgical solutions should be subsequently performed. Corneal opacities may result from chlorine solution being sprayed into the eyes.

For decontaminating fabric clothing or equipment, a 5% hypochlorite solution should be used, although many fabrics will be damaged with this concentration of hypochlorite. For decontaminating equipment, a contact time of 30 min before normal cleaning is required. This is corrosive to most metals and injurious to most fabrics, so rinse thoroughly and oil metal surfaces after completion.

Bio-agents may be rendered harmless through such physical means as heat and radiation. Agents are rendered completely harmless by sterilization with dry heat for 2 h at 160°C. If autoclaving with steam at 121°C and 1 atmosphere of overpressure (15 psi), the time may be reduced to 20 min, depending on volume. Solar UV radiation has a disinfectant effect, often in combination with drying. This is effective in certain environmental conditions but is hard to standardize for practical usage for decontamination purposes.

The health hazards of environmental contamination by bio-agents differ from those of persistent or volatile chemical agents. Aerosolized particles in the 1-5 m size range will remain suspended by brownian motion and can disseminate widely. Suspended bio-agents would be eventually inactivated by solar UV light, desiccation, and oxidation. Little, if any environmental residues would remain. Possible exceptions include residue near the dissemination line or in the immediate area surrounding point-source munitions. Bio-agents deposited on the soil would be subject to degradation by environmental stressors and competing soil microflora. Simulant studies suggest that secondary reaerosolization would be difficult, but may pose a human health hazard. Environmental decontamination of terrain is costly and difficult. If grossly contaminated terrain, streets, or roads must be passed, the use of dust-binding spray to minimize reaerosolization may be considered. If it is necessary to decontaminate these surfaces, chlorine-calcium or lye may be used. Otherwise, rely on the natural processes that, especially outdoors, lead to the decontamination of agent by drying and solar UV radiation. Rooms in fixed spaces are best decontaminated with aerosolized gases or liquids (e.g., formaldehyde). This is usually combined with surface disinfectants to ensure complete effectiveness.

For further information on decontamination, see FM 3-5, *NBC Decontamination*; FM 4-02.7, *Health Service Support in a NBC Environment*; and Army FM 8-284, *Treatment of Biological Warfare Agent Casualties.*

Electronic copies of all DoD publications are available at the Defense Technical Information Center (DTIC), http://www.dtic.mil/ dtic.

APPENDICES

APPENDIX A: LIST OF MEDICAL TERMS & ACRONYMS

Partly adapted from:
Stedman's Electronic Medical Dictionary,
Williams & Wilkins, Baltimore, MD, 2006,
Principles and Practice of Infectious Diseases, and
Mandell et al, 7th Edition.

Acetylcholine (ACH, Ach) - The neurotransmitter substance at cholinergic synapses, which causes cardiac inhibition, vasodilation, gastrointestinal peristalsis, and other parasympathetic effects. It is liberated from preganglionic and postganglionic endings of parasympathetic fibers and from preganglionic fibers of the sympathetic as a result of nerve injuries, whereupon it acts as a transmitter on the effector organ; it is hydrolyzed into choline and acetic acid by acetylcholinesterase before a second impulse may be transmitted.

ACIP - Advisory Committee on Immunization Practices; Overseen by the CDC.

Active vaccination -The act of artificially stimulating the body to develop antibodies against infectious disease by the administration of vaccines or toxoids.

Adenopathy - Swelling or morbid enlargement of the lymph nodes.

AHF - Argentine hemorrhagic fever, a VHF.

AIDS - Acquired Immunodeficiency Syndrome.

Aleukia - Absence or extremely decreased number of leukocytes in the circulating blood.

ALT - Alanine aminotransferase, a liver enzyme.

Analgesic - 1. A compound capable of producing analgesia, i.e., one that relieves pain by altering perception of nociceptive stimuli without producing anesthesia or loss of consciousness. 2. Characterized by reduced response to painful stimuli.

Anaphylaxis - The term is commonly used to denote the immediate, transient kind of immunologic (allergic) reaction characterized by contraction of smooth muscle and dilation of capillaries due to release of pharmacologically active substances (histamine, bradykinin, serotonin, and slow-reacting substance), classically initiated by the combination of antigen (allergen) with mast cell-fixed, cytophilic antibody (chiefly IgE).

Anticonvulsant - An agent that prevents or arrests seizures.

Antigen - Any substance that, as a result of coming in contact with appropriate cells, induces a state of sensitivity or immune responsiveness and that reacts in a demonstrable way with antibodies or immune cells of the sensitized subject in vivo or in vitro.

Antitoxin - An antibody formed in response to and capable of neutralizing a biological poison; a serum prepared from animals vaccinated against a specific toxin.

ARDS - Acute Respiratory Distress Syndrome

Arthralgia - Severe pain in a joint, especially one not inflammatory in character.

AST - Aspartate aminotransferase, a liver enzyme.

Asthenia - Weakness or debility.

Ataxia - An inability to coordinate muscle activity during voluntary movement, so that smooth movements occur. Most often due to disorders of the cerebellum or the posterior columns of the spinal cord; may involve the limbs, head, or trunk.

Atelectasis - Decrease or loss of air in all or part of the lung, with resulting loss of lung volume itself.

ATLS - Advanced Trauma Life Support.

Atropine - An anticholinergic, with diverse effects (tachycardia, mydriasis, cycloplegia, constipation, urinary retention) attributable to reversible competitive blockade of acetylcholine at muscarinic type cholinergic receptors; used in the treatment of poisoning with organophosphate insecticides or nerve gases.

ASAP - As soon as possible.

AVA - Anthrax Vaccine Adsorbed.

BDO- Battle dress overgarment.

BHF - Bolivian Hemorrhagic Fever, a VHF.

BID or bid- Twice each day.

Bilirubin - A yellow bile pigment formed from hemoglobin during normal and abnormal destruction of erythrocytes. Excess bilirubin is associated with jaundice.

Bio-agent – Biological agent; biological threat agent.

Blood agar - A mixture of blood and nutrient agar used for the cultivation of many medically important microorganisms.

BMR - Biological response modifier.

BoNT - Botulinum neurotoxin.

Bronchiolitis - Inflammation of the bronchioles often associated with bronchopneumonia.

Bronchitis - Inflammation of the mucous membrane of the bronchi.

Brucella - A genus of encapsulated, nonmotile bacteria (family Brucellaceae) containing short, rod-shaped to coccoid, gram-negative cells. These organisms are parasitic, invading all animal tissues and causing infection of the genital organs, the mammary gland, and the respiratory and intestinal tracts, and are pathogenic for humans and various species of domestic animals. They do not produce gas from carbohydrates.

BSL - Bio-safety level.

BTRP - Biological Threat Reduction Program.

Bubo - Inflammatory swelling of one or more lymph nodes, usually in the groin; the confluent mass of nodes usually suppurates and drains pus.

Bulla, gen. and pl. bullae - A large blister greater than 1 cm in diameter appearing as a circumscribed area of separation of the epidermis from the subepidermal structure (subepidermal *bulla*) or as a circumscribed area of separation of epidermal cells (intraepidermal *bulla*) caused by the presence of serum, or occasionally by an injected substance.

BW - Biological Warfare.

Carbuncle - Deep-seated pyogenic infection of the skin and subcutaneous tissues, usually arising in several contiguous hair follicles, with formation of connecting sinuses; often preceded or accompanied by fever, malaise, and prostration.

Case Fatality Rate (CFR) - The proportion or percentage of deaths within a designated population of people with a particular disease, over the course of the disease. (*Cf.* mortality rate.)

CBC - Complete blood count.

CBDP - The DoD's Chemical and Biological Defense Program.

CBEP - Cooperative Biological Engagement Program.

CBRN(E) - Chemical, biological, radiological, and nuclear (and explosives).

CCHF - Congo-Crimean hemorrhagic fever, a VHF.

CDC - United States Centers for Disease Control and Prevention, Atlanta, Georgia.

Cerebrospinal - Relating to the brain and the spinal cord.

CF - Complement fixation.

CFR - Case Fatality Rate (*q.v.*).

Chemoprophylaxis - Prevention of disease by the use of chemicals or drugs.

Cholinergic - Relating to nerve cells or fibers that employ acetylcholine as their neurotransmitter.

Cm(s) - Centimeter(s)

CNS - Central nervous system.

Coagulopathy - A disease affecting the coagulability of the blood.

Coccobacillus - A short, thick bacterial rod of the shape of an oval or slightly elongated coccus.

Conjunctiva, pl. conjunctivae - The mucous membrane investing the anterior surface of the eyeball and the posterior surface of the lids.

CPO - Chemical protective overgarment.

CPT - Current Procedural Terminology; maintained by the American Medical Association.

CSF - Cerebrospinal fluid.

CTR - DTRA's Cooperative Threat Reduction program.

Cutaneous - Relating to the skin.

CW - Chemical warfare.

CXR - Chest X-ray

Cyanosis - A dark bluish or purplish coloration of the skin and mucous membrane due to deficient oxygenation of the blood, evident when reduced hemoglobin in the blood exceeds 5 g per 100 ml.

D - Day(s)

DARPA - Defense Advanced Research Projects Agency.

DHHS - United States Department of Health and Human Services; Oversees FDA, CDC, etc.

DHS - United States Department of Homeland Security.

Diathesis -The constitutional or inborn state disposing to a disease, group of diseases, or metabolic or structural anomaly.

Diplopia -The condition in which a single object is perceived as two objects. SYN: double vision.

Distal - Situated away from the center of the body, or from the point of origin; specifically applied to the extremity or distant part of a limb or organ.

DNA - Deoxyribonucleic Acid

DoD - United States Department of Defense.

DTRA - The DoD's Defense Threat Reduction Agency.

DVD - Digital versatile disc or digital videodisk.

Dysarthria - A disturbance of speech and language due to emotional stress, to brain injury, or to paralysis, incoordination, or spasticity of the muscles used for speaking.

Dysphagia, dysphagy - Difficulty in swallowing.

Dysphonia - Altered voice production.

Dyspnea - Shortness of breath, a subjective difficulty or distress in breathing, usually associated with disease of the heart or lungs; occurs normally during intense physical exertion or at high altitude.

Ecchymosis - A purplish patch caused by extravasation of blood into the skin, differing from petechiae only in size (larger than 3 mm diameter).

ECL - Electrochemiluminescence.

EDP - Especially Dangerous Pathogen(s)

EIND - Emergency IND.

Electrochemiluminescence - A method used to identify microorganisms. It is a relatively new technique for this purpose and is similar in operation to ELISA, FA and sandwich antibody assays. A capture antibody bound to a magnetic bead captures the target microorganism. Another antibody labeled with a ruthenium tris-bipyridyl compound ($Ru(bpy)_3^{2+}$) is introduced. A magnet is used to pull the beads to an electrode which is used to excite the ruthenium compound which then emits light. The light is detected revealing the presences of the target organism. The method is easily automated and is generally faster than either ELISA or FA.

EO - Executive Order

Eczema - Generic term for inflammatory conditions of the skin, particularly with vesiculation in the acute stage, typically erythematous, edematous, papular, and crusting; followed often by lichenification and scaling and occasionally by duskiness of the erythema and, infrequently, hyperpigmentation; often accompanied by sensations of itching and burning.

ED_{50} - Median effective dose; the dose that produces the desired effect; when followed by a subscript (generally "ED_{50}"), it denotes the dose having such an effect on a certain percentage (e.g., 50%) of the test animals.

Edema - An accumulation of an excessive amount of watery fluid in cells, tissues, or serous cavities.

EEE - Eastern Equine Encephalitis [virus]

ELISA - Enzyme-linked immunosorbent assay (*q.v.*).

Enanthem, enanthema - A mucous membrane eruption, especially one occurring in connection with one of the exanthemas.

Encephalitis, pl. encephalitides - Inflammation of the brain.

Endotoxemia - Presence in the blood of endotoxins.

Endotracheal intubation - Passage of a tube through the nose or mouth into the trachea for maintenance of the airway during anesthesia or for maintenance of an imperiled airway.

Enterotoxin - A cytotoxin specific for the cells of the intestinal mucosa.

Enzyme-Linked Immunosorbent Assay - A method used to detect a microbial antigen or an antibody to a microbial antigen. It works by chemically linking an enzyme to an antibody that recognizes and adheres to the desired antigen or antibody. Any unbound antibody-enzyme complex is removed. A chemical that is converted by the enzyme into a fluorescent compound is applied and allowed to react. The fluorescence is then detected to reveal the presence or absence of the antigen or antibody.

Epistaxis - Profuse bleeding from the nose.

Epizootic - 1. Denoting a temporal pattern of disease occurrence in an animal population in which the disease occurs with a frequency clearly in excess of the expected frequency in that population during a given time interval. 2. An outbreak (epidemic) of disease in an animal population; often with the implication that it may also affect human populations.

Erythema - Redness of the skin due to capillary dilatation.

Erythema multiforme - An acute eruption of macules, papules, or subdermal vesicles presenting a multiform appearance, the characteristic lesion being the target or iris lesion over the dorsal aspect of the hands and forearms; its origin may be allergic, seasonal, or from drug sensitivity, and the eruption, although usually self-limited (e.g., multiforme minor), may be recurrent or may run a severe course, sometimes with fatal termination (e.g., multiforme major or Stevens-Johnson syndrome).

Erythrocyte - A mature red blood cell.

Erythropoiesis - The formation of red blood cells.

EUA - Emergency Use Authorization

Exanthema - A skin eruption occurring as a symptom of an acute viral or coccal disease, as in scarlet fever or measles.

Extracellular - Outside the cells.

Extraocular - Adjacent to but outside the eyeball.

FA - Fluorescent antibody (*q.v.*).

FAC - free available chlorine.

Fasciculation - Involuntary contractions, or twitchings, of groups (fasciculi) of muscle fibers, a coarser form of muscular contraction than fibrillation.

FBI - United States Federal Bureau of Investigation

FDA - United States Food and Drug Administration; Part of DHHS.

Febrile - Denoting or relating to fever.

FEMA - Federal Emergency Management Agency

FM - Field Manual

Fomite - Objects, such as clothing, towels, and utensils that possibly harbor a disease agent and are capable of transmitting it.

Formalin - A 37% aqueous solution of formaldehyde.

Fluorescent antibody - A method used in microbiology to detect microorganisms usually bacteria. An antibody with an attached fluorescent molecule is applied to a slide containing the bacteria and washed to remove unbound antibody. Under UV light the bacteria to which antibodies are bound will fluoresce, revealing their presence

Fulminant hepatitis - Severe, rapidly progressive loss of hepatic function due to viral infection or other cause of inflammatory destruction of liver tissue with associated coagulopathy and encephalopathy.

Generalized vaccinia - Secondary lesions of the skin after vaccination, which may occur in subjects with previously healthy skin but are more common in the case of traumatized skin, especially in the case of eczema (eczema vaccinatum). In the latter instance, generalized vaccinia may result from mere contact with a vaccinated person. Secondary vaccinial lesions may also occur after transfer of virus from the vaccination to another site by means of the fingers (autoinoculation).

GI - Gastrointestinal

Glanders - A chronic debilitating disease of horses and other equids, as well as some members of the cat family, caused by *Pseudomonas mallei*; it is transmissible to humans. It attacks the mucous membranes of the nostrils of the horse, producing an increased and vitiated secretion and discharge of mucus, and enlargement and induration of the glands of the lower jaw.

Gm - Gram(s)

Granulocytopenia - Less than the normal number of granular leukocytes in the blood.

Guarnieri bodies - Intracytoplasmic acidophilic inclusion bodies observed in epithelial cells in variola (smallpox) and vaccinia infections, and which include aggregations of Paschen body's or virus particles.

H or h - Hour(s)

Hemagglutination - The agglutination of red blood cells; may be immune as a result of specific antibody either for red blood cell antigens per se or other antigens that coat the red blood cells, or may be nonimmune,,as in hemagglutination caused by viruses or other microbes.

Hemagglutinin - A substance, antibody or other, that causes hemagglutination.

Hematemesis - Vomiting of blood.

Hemopoietic - Pertaining to or related to the formation of blood cells.

Hematuria - Any condition in which the urine contains blood or red blood cells.

Hemodynamic - Relating to the physical aspects of the blood circulation.

Hemolysis - Alteration, dissolution, or destruction of red blood cells in such a manner that hemoglobin is liberated into the medium in which the cells are suspended, e.g., by specific complement-fixing antibodies, toxins, various chemical agents, tonicity, alteration of temperature.

Hemolytic Uremic Syndrome - Hemolytic anemia and thrombocytopenia occurring with acute renal failure.

Hemoptysis - The spitting of blood derived from the lungs or bronchial tubes as a result of pulmonary or bronchial hemorrhage.

HEPA - High-Efficiency Particulate Air [filter]

Hepatic - Relating to the liver.

Heterologous - 1. Pertaining to cytologic or histologic elements occurring where they are not normally found. 2. Derived from an animal of a different species, as the serum of a horse is heterologous for a rabbit.

HFRS - Hemorrhagic fever with renal syndrome. A viral hemorrhagic fever syndrome caused by viruses of the genus *Hantavirus*, Bunyaviridae family, with renal impairment as the primary organ manifestation.

Hyperemia - The presence of an increased amount of blood in a part or organ.

Hyperesthesia - Abnormal acuteness of sensitivity to touch, pain, or other sensory stimuli.

Hypotension - Subnormal arterial blood pressure.

Hypovolemia - A decreased amount of blood in the body.

Hypoxemia - Subnormal oxygenation of arterial blood, short of anoxia.

IA - Inhalational anthrax.

Idiopathic - Denoting a disease of unknown cause.

ICD - International Classification of Diseases; published by the WHO.

ICLC - Interstitial Cajal-like cells.

IHR - International Health Regulations.

IM - Intramuscular; intramuscularly.

Immunoassay - Detection and assay of substances by serological (immunological) methods; in most applications the substance in question serves as antigen, both in antibody production and in measurement of antibody by the test substance.

In vitro - In an artificial environment, referring to a process or reaction occurring therein, as in a test tube or culture medium.

In vivo - In the living body, referring to a process or reaction occurring therein.

IND – Investigational New Drug; FDA's terminology for an experimental drug or vaccine, not approved for general use.

Induration - 1. The process of becoming extremely firm or hard, or having such physical features. 2. A focus or region of indurated tissue.

Inguinal - Relating to the groin.

Inoculation - Introduction of the causative organism of a disease into the body.

IV - Intravenous; intravenously.

JPEO-CBD - The DoD's Joint Program Executive Office for Chemical and Biological Defense.

JSGPM - Joint Service General Protective Mask (U.S. Army XM-50).

JSLIST - Joint Services Lightweight Integrated Suit Technology.

Kg - Kilogram(s).

KGB - The USSR's "Committee for State Security" [*Komitet gosudarstvennoy bezopasnosti*].

LD_{50} - In toxicology, the LD'_{50} of a particular substance is a measure of how much constitutes a lethal dose. In toxicological studies of substances, one test is to administer varying doses of the substance to populations of test animals; that dose administered which kills half the test population is referred to as the LD_{50}

LDH - lactate dehydrogenase, a liver enzyme.

Leukopenia - The antithesis of leukocytosis; any situation in which the total number of leukocytes in the circulating blood is less than normal, the lower limit of which is generally regarded as 4000-5000 per cubic mm.

LRN - Laboratory Response Network

Lumbosacral - Relating to the lumbar vertebrae and the sacrum.

Lumen, pl. lumina - The space in the interior of a tubular structure, such as an artery or the intestine.

Lymphadenopathy - Any disease process affecting a lymph node or lymph nodes.

Lymphopenia - A reduction, relative or absolute, in the number of lymphocytes in the circulating blood.

Macula, pl. maculae - 1. A small spot, perceptibly different in color from the surrounding tissue. 2. A small, discolored patch or spot on the skin, neither elevated above nor depressed below the skin's surface.

Mediastinitis - Inflammation of the cellular tissue of the mediastinum.

Mediastinum - The median partition of the thoracic cavity, covered by the mediastinal pleura and containing all the thoracic viscera and structures except the lungs.

MCM - Medical countermeasure.

Megakaryocyte - A large cell with a polyploid nucleus that is usually multilobed; megakaryocytes are normally present in bone marrow, not in the circulating blood, and give rise to blood platelets.

Melena - Passage of dark-colored, tarry stools, due to the presence of blood altered by the intestinal juices.

Meningism - A condition in which the symptoms simulate a meningitis, but in which no actual inflammation of these membranes is present.

Meningococcemia - Presence of meningococci (*N. meningitidis*) in the circulating blood.

Meninges - Any membrane; specifically, one of the membranous coverings of the brain and spinal cord.

Microcyst - A tiny cyst, frequently of such dimensions that a magnifying lens or microscope is required for observation.

Microscopy - Investigation of minute objects by means of a microscope.

Min - Minute(s)

MOPP - Mission Oriented Protective Posture; U.S. Army terminology for NBC protective gear.

Mo(s) - Month(s)

Mortality rate - A measure of the number of deaths (in general, or due to a specific cause) in some population, scaled to the size of that population, per unit time. (*Cf.* Case fatality rate)

Mg - Milligram(s)

Moribund - Dying; at the point of death.

Mucocutaneous - Relating to mucous membrane and skin; denoting the line of junction of the two at the nasal, oral, vaginal, and anal orifices.

MULO - Multipurpose rain/snow/CW overboots.

Myalgia - Muscular pain.

Mydriasis - Dilation of the pupil.

NATO - North Atlantic Treaty Organization.

NBC - Nuclear, Biological and Chemical

Narcosis - General and nonspecific reversible depression of neuronal excitability, produced by a number of physical and chemical agents, usually resulting in stupor rather than in anesthesia.

Necrosis - Pathologic death of one or more cells, or of a portion of tissue or organ, resulting from irreversible damage.

Nephropathia epidemica - A generally benign form of epidemic hemorrhagic fever reported in Scandinavia.

Neutrophilia - An increase of neutrophilic leukocytes in blood or tissues; also frequently used synonymously with leukocytosis, inasmuch as the latter is generally the result of an increased number of neutrophilic granulocytes in the circulating blood (or in the tissues, or both).

Nosocomial - Denoting a new disorder (not the patient's original condition) associated with being treated in a hospital, such as a hospital-acquired infection.

ODP - Office of Domestic Preparedness; Overseen by both the U.S. Department of Justice and DHS.

Oliguria - Scant urine production.

Oropharynx - The portion of the pharynx that lies posterior to the mouth; it is continuous above with the nasopharynx via the pharyngeal isthmus and below with the laryngopharynx.

Osteomyelitis - Inflammation of the bone marrow and adjacent bone.

Pancytopenia - Pronounced reduction in the number of erythrocytes, all types of white blood cells, and the blood platelets in the circulating blood.

Pandemic - Denoting a disease affecting or attacking the population of an extensive region, country, continent; extensively epidemic.

PAPR - Powered air-purifying respirator.

Papule - A small, circumscribed, solid elevation up to 1 cm in diameter on the skin.

Parasitemia -The presence of parasites in the circulating blood; used especially with reference to malarial and other protozoan forms, and microfilariae.

Passive immunity - Providing temporary protection from disease through the administration of exogenously produced antibody (i.e., transplacental transmission of antibodies to the fetus or the injection of immune globulin for specific preventive purposes).

PCR - Polymerase chain reaction (*q.v.*).

PEP - Post-exposure prophylaxis

Percutaneous - Denoting the passage of substances through unbroken skin, for example, by needle puncture, including introduction of wires and catheters.

Perivascular - Surrounding a blood or lymph vessel.

Petechia, pl. petechiae - Minute hemorrhagic spots, of pinpoint to pinhead size, in the skin, which are not blanched by pressure.

Pharyngeal - Relating to the pharynx.

Pharyngitis - Inflammation of the mucous membrane and underlying parts of the pharynx.

Phosgene - Carbonyl chloride; a colorless liquid below 8.2°C, but an extremely poisonous gas at ordinary temperatures; it is an insidious gas, as it is not immediately irritating, even when fatal concentrations are inhaled.

Photophobia - Light-induced pain, especially of the eyes; for example, in uveitis, the light-induced movement of the iris may be painful. SYN: photodynia, photalgia

Pleurisy - Inflammation of the pleura.

PO – By mouth; orally

Polymerase chain reaction (PCR) - An in vitro method for enzymatically synthesizing and amplifying defined sequences of DNA in molecular biology. Can be used for improving DNA-based diagnostic procedures for identifying unknown biowarfare agents.

Polymorphonuclear - Having nuclei of varied forms; denoting a variety of leukocyte.

Polyuria - Excessive excretion of urine.

PPE - Personal protective equipment.

Presynaptic - Pertaining to the area on the proximal side of a synaptic cleft.

Prophylaxis, pl. prophylaxes - Prevention of disease or of a process that can lead to disease.

Prostration - A marked loss of strength, as in exhaustion.

Proteinuria - Presence of urinary protein in concentrations greater than 0.3 g in a 24-hour urine collection or in concentrations greater than 1 g/l in a random urine collection on two or more occasions at least 6 hours apart; specimens must be clean, voided midstream, or obtained by catheterization.

Pruritus - Syn: itching.

Ptosis, pl. ptoses - In reference to the eyes, drooping of the eyelids.

Pulmonary edema - Edema of the lungs.

Pyrogenic - Causing fever.

QD or qD - Each day

QID or qid – Four times each day

Retinitis - Inflammation of the retina.

Retrosternal - Posterior to the sternum.

Rhinorrhea - A discharge from the nasal mucous membrane.

RNA - Ribonucleic Acid.

RT - Reverse transcriptase.

RVF –Rift Valley fever, a VHF.

SAHF - South American Hemorrhagic Fever (includes AHF, BHF)

Sarin - A nerve poison which is a very potent irreversible cholinesterase inhibitor and a more toxic nerve gas than tabun or soman.

SARS - Severe Acute Respiratory Syndrome [virus].

Scarification -The making of a number of superficial incisions in the skin. It is the technique used to administer tularemia and smallpox vaccines.

Scud – NATO reporting name (SS-1 Scud) for a series of tactical ballistic missiles developed by the USSR and exported widely to other countries, including Iraq.

SEB - Staphylococcal Enterotoxin B

Septic shock - 1. Shock associated with sepsis, usually associated with abdominal and pelvic infection complicating trauma or operations; 2. Shock associated with septicemia caused by gram-negative bacteria.

Sequela, pl. sequelae - A condition after a consequence of a disease.

Shigellosis - Bacillary dysentery caused by bacteria of the genus *Shigella*, often occurring in epidemic patterns.

SNS - Strategic National Stockpile; Repository of drugs, vaccines, etc, overseen jointly by CDC and DHS.

Soman - An extremely potent cholinesterase inhibitor, similar to sarin and tabun.

Sterile abscess - An abscess whose contents are not caused by pyogenic bacteria.

Stridor - A high-pitched, noisy respiration, like the blowing of the wind; a sign of respiratory obstruction, especially in the trachea or larynx.

Superantigen - An antigen that interacts with the T-cell receptor in a domain outside of the antigen recognition site. This type of interaction induces the activation of larger numbers of T cells compared to antigens that are presented in the antigen-recognition site leading to the release of numerous cytokines.

Superinfection - A new infection in addition to one already present.

Tachycardia - Rapid beating of the heart, conventionally applied to rates over 100 per minute.

Teratogenicity - The property or capability of producing fetal malformation.

Thrombocytopenia - A condition in which there is an abnormally small number of platelets in the circulating blood.

TID or tid - Thrice each day

TMP-SMX - Trimethoprim-sulfamethoxazole

Toxoid - A modified bacterial toxin that has been rendered nontoxic (commonly with formaldehyde) but retains the ability to stimulate the formation of antitoxins (antibodies) and thus producing an active immunity. Examples include botulinum, tetanus, and diphtheria toxoids.

Tracheitis - Inflammation of the lining membrane of the trachea.

Urticaria - An eruption of itching wheals, usually of systemic origin; it may be due to a state of hypersensitivity to foods or drugs, foci of infection, physical agents (heat, cold, light, friction), or psychic stimuli.

USAMRICD – United States Army Medical Research Institute of Chemical Defense, Aberdeen Proving Ground, Maryland.

USAMRIID – United States Army Medical Research Institute of Infectious Diseases, Fort Detrick, Maryland.

UK - United Kingdom

UN - United Nations

USSR - Union of Soviet Socialist Republics

UV - Ultraviolet

Vaccine - A suspension of attenuated live or killed microorganisms (bacteria, viruses, or rickettsiae), or fractions thereof (for example, specific protein subunits or naked DNA), administered to induce immunity and thereby prevent infectious disease.

Vaccinia - An infection, primarily local and limited to the site of inoculation, induced in humans by inoculation with the vaccinia (coxpox) virus to confer resistance to smallpox (variola). On about the third day after vaccination, papules form at the site of inoculation which become transformed into umbilicated vesicles and later pustules; they then dry up, and the scab falls off on about the 21st day, leaving a pitted scar. In some cases there are more or less marked constitutional disturbances.

Varicella - An acute contagious disease, usually occurring in children, caused by the varicella-zoster virus, a member of the family *Herpesviridae*, and marked by a sparse eruption of papules, which become vesicles and then pustules, like that of smallpox although less severe and varying in stages, usually with mild constitutional symptoms; incubation period is about 14 to 17 days. Syn: chickenpox

Variola - Syn: smallpox.

Variolation - The historical practice of inducing immunity against smallpox by inoculating the skin with matter from skin pustules of a smallpox victim. Said to have first been done in China about 1022 B.C.

VEE - Venezuelan Equine Encephalitis [virus].

VHF - Viral Hemorrhagic Fever.

Viremia - The presence of virus in the bloodstream.

Virion - The complete virus particle that is structurally intact and infectious.

WEE - Western Equine Encephalitis [virus]

Wk(s) - Week(s)

WMD - Weapon(s) of Mass Destruction; see also NBC.

WHO - The UN's World Health Organization.

Zoonosis - An infection or infestation shared in nature by humans and other animals that are the normal or usual host; a disease of humans acquired from an animal source.

APPENDIX B: PATIENT ISOLATION PRECAUTIONS

STANDARD PRECAUTIONS:

(Standard precautions should be applied to all patients in a healthcare setting regardless of the suspected or confirmed presence of an infectious agent.)

- Wash hands with soap and water or use alcohol-based sanitizer before and after patient contact and between patients.
- Wear gloves when touching blood, body fluids, secretions, excretions, and contaminated items.
- Wear a mask and eye protection, or a face shield during procedures likely to generate splashes or sprays of blood, body fluids, secretions or excretions
- Handle used patient-care equipment and linen in a manner that prevents the transfer of microorganisms to people or equipment.
- Use safe injection practices.
- Use respiratory hygiene / cough etiquette.

Use a mouthpiece or other ventilation device as an alternative to mouth-to-mouth resuscitation when practical.

<u>Standard precautions are employed in the care of ALL patients</u>

TRANSMISSION-BASED PRECAUTIONS

(The following transmission-based precautions are used in combination with standard precautions when prolonged viability of a specific organism or toxin is known or suspected on unknown agent. Multiple transmission-based precautions may be used related to the agent if multiple routes of transmission occur.)

CONTACT PRECAUTIONS

Standard Precautions plus

- Place the patient in a private room or cohort them with someone with the same infection if possible; $\geq$3 feet spatial separation
- Wear a gown and gloves when entering the room if contact with patient is anticipated or other surfaces patient has touched especially if patient has diarrhea, a colostomy or wound drainage not covered by a dressing.

- Don personal protective equipment (PPE) upon room entry and discard before exiting the patient room to contain pathogens. Change gloves after contact with infective material.
- Limit the movement or transport of the patient from the room and if needed, lightly cover open wounds for transport.
- Ensure that patient-care items, bedside equipment, and frequently touched surfaces receive daily cleaning.
- Dedicate use of noncritical patient-care equipment (such as stethoscopes) to a single patient, or cohort patients with the same pathogen. Use single-use/ disposable equipment if possible. If not feasible, adequate disinfection between patients is necessary.

Conventional Diseases requiring Contact Precautions: MRSA, VRE, Clostridium difficile, RSV, enteroviruses, enteric infections in the incontinent host, skin infections (SSSS, HSV, impetigo, lice, scabies), hemorrhagic conjunctivitis.

Biothreat Diseases requiring Contact Precautions: Viral Hemorrhagic Fevers. Smallpox

DROPLET PRECAUTIONS

Standard Precaution plus

- Place the patient in a private room or cohort them with someone with the same infection. If not feasible, maintain at least 3 feet between patients.
- Wear a surgical mask when working within 3 feet of the patient.
- Limit movement and transport of the patient. Place a mask on the patient if tolerated and they need to be moved.

Conventional Diseases Requiring Droplet Precautions: Invasive *Haemophilus influenzae* and meningococcal disease, drug-resistant pneumococcal disease, diphtheria, pertussis, mycoplasma, GABHS, influenza, mumps, rubella, parvovirus.

Biothreat Diseases Requiring Droplet precautions: Pneumonic Plague

AIRBORNE PRECAUTIONS

Standard Precautions plus:

- Place the patient in a private room that has monitored negative air pressure, a minimum of six air changes/hour, and appropriate filtration of air before it is exhausted directly to outside or HEPA filtration before discharged from the room.

- Wear respiratory protection when entering the room. N95 or higher masks are effective against particulates 1-5 micrometers in size.
- Limit movement and transport of the patient. Place a mask on the patient if they need to be moved. DO NOT place N95 mask or higher on patient who has trouble inhaling. Utilize a standard surgical mask.

Conventional Diseases Requiring Airborne Precautions: Measles, Varicella, Pulmonary Tuberculosis.

Biothreat Diseases Requiring Airborne Precautions: Smallpox.

Discontinuation of Transmission Based Precautions: One or more transmission-based precautions can be discontinued when patient is not infectious and no longer requires them or the related disease is ruled out as a diagnosis. Each disease differs on when to specifically discontinue use. Standard precautions will be used, however, even after all related transmission-based precautions have been removed.

For more information, see: Siegel JD, Rhinehart E, Jackson M, Chiarello L, and the Healthcare Infection Control Practices Advisory Committee, 2007 Guideline for Isolation Precautions: Preventing Transmission of Infectious Agents in Healthcare Settings **http://www.cdc.gov/ncidod/dhqp/pdf/isolation2007.pdf**

APPENDIX C: BIOAGENT CHARACTERISTICS

Disease	Transmit Human to Human	Infective Dose (Aerosol)/LD_{50} *1	Incubation Period
Anthrax	No	8,000-50,000 spores	1-6 days
Brucellosis	No	10 -100 organisms	5-60 days (usually 1-2 months)
Glanders	Low	Unknown, Potentially low	10-14 days via aerosol
Melioidosis	Low	Unknown, Potentially low	1-21 days (up to years)
Plague	Moderate, Pneumonic	500–15000 organisms	1-7 days (usually 2-3 days)
Tularemia	No	10-50 organisms	1-21 days (average 3-6)
Q Fever	Rare	1-10 organisms	7-41 days
Smallpox	High	Assumed low (10-100) organisms)	7-17 days (average 12)
Venezuelan Equine Encephalitis	Rare	10-100 organisms	2-6 days
Viral Hemorrhagic Fevers	Moderate	1-10 organisms	4-21 days
Botulism	No	0.001 μmg/kg is LD_{50} for type A (parenteral), 0.003 μmg/kg (aerosol)	12 hours -5 days
Staph Enterotoxin B	No	0.03 μmg / person (80kg) incapacitation	3-12 hours after inhalation
Ricin	No	3-5 mg/kg is LD_{50} in mice	18-24 hours
T-2 Mycotoxins	No	Moderate	2-4 hours

*1 In this Table, Infective Dose is representative of bacteria and viruses, while LD50 is representative of toxins

Duration of Illness	Lethality (approx. case fatality rates)	Persistence of Organism	Vaccine Efficacy (aerosol exposure)
3-5 days (usually fatal if untreated)	High	Very stable–spores remain viable for > 40 years in soil	2 dose efficacy against up to 1,000 LD_{50} in monkeys
Weeks to months	<5% untreated	Very stable	No vaccine
Death in 7-10 days in septicemic form	> 50%	Very stable	No vaccine
Death in 2-3 days with septicemic form (untreated)	19– 50% for severe disease	Very stable; survives indefinitely in warm moist soil or stagnant water	No vaccine
1-6 days (usually fatal)	High unless treated within 12-24 hours	For up to 1 year in soil; 270 days in live tissue	No vaccine
≥ 2 weeks	Moderate if untreated	For months in moist soil or other media	80% protection against 1-10 LD_{50}
2-14 days	Very low	For months on wood and sand	94% protection against 3,500 LD_{50} in guinea pigs
4 weeks	High to moderate	Very stable	Vaccine protects against large doses in primates
Days to weeks	Low	Relatively unstable	TC 83 protects against 30-500 LD_{50} in hamsters
Death between 7-16 days	High to moderate depends on agent	Relatively unstable–depends on agent	No vaccine
Death in 24-72 hours; lasts months if not lethal	High without respiratory support	For weeks in nonmoving water and food	3 dose efficacy 100% against 25-250 LD_{50} in primates
Hours	< 1%	Resistant to freezing	No vaccine
Days–death within 10-12 days for ingestion	High	Stable	No vaccine
Days to months	Moderate	For years at room temp Tt	No vaccine

APPENDIX D: BIOAGENT PROPHYLACTICS & THERAPEUTICS

ANTHRAX

VACCINE/TOXOID

Bioport BioThrax™ Anthrax Vaccine (AVA)

Preexposure [A]: licensed for adults 18-65-yr old, 0.5 mL IM @ 0, 2, 4 wk, 6, 12, 18 mo then annual boosters

Postexposure [IND]: DoD Contingency Use Protocol for volunteer anthrax vaccination SQ @ 0, 2, 4 wk in combination with approved and labeled antibiotics

Pediatric Annex [IND] for postexposure use.

http://www.anthrax.osd.mil/resource/policies/policies.asp

CHEMOPROPHYLAXIS

N.B. - 60 days postexposure prophylaxis recommended regardless of full or partial vaccination (FM 8-284)

After a suspected exposure to aerosolized anthrax of unknown antibiotic susceptibility, prophylaxis with ciprofloxacin (500 mg PO bid for adults, and 10-15 mg/kg po bid (up to 1 g/day) for children) OR doxycycline (100 mg PO bid for adults or children >8 yr and >45 kg, and 2.2 mg/kg PO bid (up to 200 mg/day) for children < 8yr) should be initiated immediately.

If antibiotic susceptibilities allow, patients who cannot tolerate tetracyclines or quinolones can be switched to amoxicillin (500 mg PO tid for adults and 80 mg/kg divided tid (≥ 1.5 g/day) in children).

The ACIP recommends a postexposure regimen of 60 days of appropriate antimicrobial prophylaxis combined with three doses administered SQ (0, 2, and 4 weeks) for previously unvaccinated persons aged >18 years. The licensed vaccination schedule can be resumed at 6 months. The first dose of vaccine should be administered within 10 days. Persons for whom vaccination has been delayed should extend antimicrobial use to 14 days after the third dose (even if this practice might result in use of antimicrobials for > 60 days).

ANTHRAX

CHEMOTHERAPY

Inhalational*, Gastrointestinal, or Systemic Cutaneous Disease:

Ciprofloxacin: 400 mg IV 1 12 h initially then by mouth (adult)[(A)]

15 mg/kg/dose (up to 400 mg/dose) q 12 h (peds)[(A)], or

Doxycycline: 200 mg IV, then 100 mg IV q 12 h (adults)[(A)]

2.2mg/kg (100mg/dose max) q 12 h (peds < 45kg)[(A)], or (if strain susceptible),

Penicillin G Procaine: 4 million units IV q 4 h (adults)[(A)]

50,000U/kg (up to 4M U) IV q 6h (peds)[(A)]

PLUS, One or two additional antibiotics with activity against anthrax. (e.g., clindamycin plus rifampin may be a good empiric choice, pending susceptibilities). Potential additional antibiotics include one or more of the following: clindamycin, rifampin, gentamicin, macrolides, vancomycin, imipenem, and chloramphenicol.

Convert from IV to oral therapy when the patient is stable, to complete at least 60 days of antibiotics.

Meningitis: Add Rifampin 20 mg/kg IV qd or Vancomycin 1 g IVq12h

***To complete at least 60 days of antibiotics if aerosol exposure to B. anthracis has occurred.**

COMMENTS

The American Committee on Immunization Practices (ACIP) recommends anthrax vaccine in a three-dose regimen (0, 2, 4 weeks) in combination with antimicrobial postexposure prophylaxis under an IND application for unvaccinated persons who have been exposed to anthrax under an IND or EUA

Penicillins should be used for anthrax treatment or prophylaxis only if the strain is demonstrated to be PCN-susceptible

According to CDC recommendations, amoxicillin prophylaxis is appropriate only after 14-21 days of fluoroquinolone or doxycycline and only for populations with contraindications to the other drugs (children, pregnancy)

Oral dosing (versus the preferred IV) may be necessary for treatment of systemic disease in a mass casualty situation

NB - At least 60 days of postexposure prophylaxis required if aerosol exposure

Cutaneous Anthrax: Antibiotics for cutaneous disease (without systemic complaints) resulting from a biowarfare attack involving biowarfare aerosols are the same as for postexposure prophylaxis. Cutaneous anthrax acquired from natural exposure could be treated with 7-10 days of antibiotics

(A) Approved for this use by the FDA
(B) (IND) Available as an investigational new drug for this indication (ie NOT an FDA-approved use)

BRUCELLOSIS

VACCINE/TOXOID

None

CHEMOPROPHYLAXIS

A human vaccine is not available. Chemoprophylaxis is not recommended after possible exposure to endemic disease. Prophylaxis should only be considered for high-risk exposure in the following situations: (1) inadvertent wound or mucous membrane exposure to infected livestock tissues and body fluids and to livestock vaccines, (2) exposure to laboratory aerosols or to secondary aerosols generated from contaminated soil particles in calving and lambing areas, (3) confirmed biowarfare exposure. **Despite extensive studies, optimal antibiotic therapy for brucellosis remains under dispute.**

CHEMOTHERAPY

Antibiotic therapy with doxycycline and rifampin (or with other medications) for 6 weeks is sufficient in most cases. More prolonged regimens may be required for patients with complications such as hepatitis, splenitis, meningoencephalitis, endocarditis, or osteomyelitis.

Inhalational, Gastrointestinal, or Systemic Cutaneous Disease

Significant infection: Doxycycline: 100 mg PO bid for 4-6 wks (adults)[A], **plus** Streptomycin 1 g IM qd for first 2-3 wks (adults)[A], or Doxycycline[A] + Gentamicin 5 mg/kg per day for 7 days (if streptomycin not available)

WHO guidelines for adults and children older than 8 y recommend rifampin (600-900 mg) and doxycycline qd for 6 weeks minimum. Treatment in children younger than 8 years requires rifampin and cotrimoxazole.

Less severe disease:

Doxycycline 100 mg PO bid for 6 wks (adults)[A], **plus**

Rifampin 600-900 mg/day PO qd for 4-6 wks (adults)[A]

Long-term (up to 6 mo) therapy for meningoencephalitis, endocarditis:

Rifampin + a tetracycline + an aminoglycoside (first 3 weeks)

COMMENTS

The CDC interim PEP recommendations for high-risk exposures to *Brucella* are: doxycycline 100 mg orally bid plus rifampin 600 mg qd orally.

Avoid monotherapy (high relapse). Relapse common for treatments less than 4-6 weeks.

GLANDERS & MELIODOSIS

VACCINE/TOXOID

None

CHEMOPROPHYLAXIS

No FDA approved prophylaxis exists. The antibiotic susceptibility pattern for B. mallei is similar to that of B. pseudomallei, with B. mallei exhibiting resistance to a number of antibiotics.

PO TMP/SMX for 14-21 days may be tried and should be given ASAP after exposure.

Ciprofloxacin or doxycyline are possible alternatives, but close patient observation must be made for relapse. May consider use of doxycycline, tetracycline, macrolides, augmentin, and quinolones in glanders and doxycycline, tetracycline, augmentin, and/or quinolones (if sensitive) in melioidosis

CHEMOTHERAPY

No FDA approved therapy exists.

Severe Disease: ceftazidime (40 mg/kg IV q 8 hours), or imipenem (15 mg/kg IV q 6 hr max 4 g/day), or meropenem (25 mg/kg IV q 8 hour, max 6 g/day), plus, TMP/SMX (TMP 8 mg/kg/day IV in four divided doses)

Continue IV therapy for at least 14 days and until patient clinically improved, then switch to oral maintenance therapy (see "mild disease" below) for ~2 months.

Melioidosis with septic shock: Consider addition of G-CSF 30 mg/day IV for 10 days.

Mild Disease:

Historic: PO doxycycline and TMP/SMX for at least 20 weeks, plus PO chloramphenicol for the first 8 weeks.

Alternative: doxycycline (100 mg po bid) plus TMP/SMX (4 mg/kg/day in two divided doses) for 20 weeks.

COMMENTS

Limited information exists about antibiotic therapy for glanders and melioidosis in humans because clinical studies examining antibiotic effectiveness *in vivo* are rare. No human data for postexposure prophylaxis exists. Natural strains of *B. mallei* respond to aminoglycosides and macrolides, while *B. pseudomallei* does not. *B. pseudomallei* exhibits resistance to diverse antibiotics, including first- and second-generation cephalosporins, penicillins, macrolides and aminoglycosides. Both B. mallei and and B. pseudomallei are sensitive to imipenem, and most strain are also susceptible to ceftazidime, ciprofloxacin and piperacillin.

Severe Disease: If ceftazidime or a carbapenem are not available, ampicillin/sulbactam or other intravenous beta-lactam/beta-lactamase inhibitor combinations may represent viable, albeit less-proven alternatives.

Mild Disease: Amoxicillin/clavulanate may be an alternative to doxycycline plus TMP/SMX, especially in pregnancy or for children <8-yr old.

(A) Approved for this use by the FDA
(IND) Available as an investigational new drug for this indication (i.e., NOT an FDA-approved use)

PLAGUE

VACCINE/TOXOID

None

CHEMOPROPHYLAXIS

Ciprofloxacin: 500 mg PO bid x 7 d (adults), 20mg/kg (up to 500 mg) PO bid (peds), or

Doxycycline: 100 mg PO q 12 h x 7 d (adults), 2.2 mg/kg (up to 100 mg) PO bid (peds), or

Tetracycline: 500 mg PO qid x 7 d (adults)

CHEMOTHERAPY

Traditionally, streptomycin, tetracycline, and doxycycline have been used for plague, and are approved by the FDA for this purpose.

Streptomycin: 1g q 12 hour IM (adults)[A], 15mg/kg/d div q 12 hour IM (up to 2 g/day)(peds)[A], or

Gentamicin: 5 mg/kg IM or IV qd or 2 mg/kg loading dose followed by 1.7 mg/kg IM or IV (adults), 2.5 mg/kg IM or IV q8h for 10 days (peds).

Alternatives: Doxycycline: 200 mg IV once then 100 mg IV bid until clinically improved, then 100 mg PO bid for total of 10-14 d (adults)[A], or ciprofloxacin: 400 mg IV q 12 hours until clinically improved then 750 mg PO bid for total 10-14 d, or chloramphenicol: 25 mg/kg IV, then 15 mg/kg qid x 14 d.

A minimum of 10 days of therapy is recommended (treat for at least 3-4 days after clinical recovery). Oral dosing (versus the preferred IV) may be necessary in a mass casualty situation.

Meningitis: add Chloramphenicol 25 mg/kg IV, then 15 mg/kg IV qid.

COMMENTS

Streptomycin is not widely available in the US and therefore is of limited utility. Although not licensed for use in treating plague, gentamicin is the consensus choice for parenteral therapy by many authorities. Reduce dosage in renal failure

Chloramphenicol is contraindicated in children less than 2 years. While Chloramphenicol is potentially an alternative for postexposure prophylaxis (25 mg/kg PO qid), oral formulations are available only outside the US

Alternate therapy or prophylaxis for susceptible strains: trimethoprim-sulfamethoxazole

Other fluoroquinolones or tetracyclines may represent viable alternatives to ciprofloxacin or doxycycline, respectively

Q FEVER

VACCINE/TOXOID

Inactivated Whole Cell Vaccine.
(Pre-exposure only): Licensed (Australian) Qvax™; IND DoD vaccine (similar to Qvax™) is available through USAMRIID for at-risk U.S. laboratory personnel.

CHEMOPROPHYLAXIS

Doxycycline: 100 mg PO bid x 5 d (adults), 2.2 mg/kg PO bid (peds), or tetracycline: 500 mg PO qid x 5d (adults); start postexposure prophylaxis 8-12 d postexposure.

CHEMOTHERAPY

Doxycycline is the first line treatment for all adults, and for children with severe illness. Treatment should be initiated whenever Q fever is suspected. Doxycycline therapy should be started again if the patient relapses.

Acute Q-fever: Doxycycline: 100 mg IV or PO q 12 h x at least 14 d (adults)(A), 2.2 mg/kg PO q 12 h (peds), or Tetracycline: 500 mg PO q 6 hr x at least 14 d

Alternatives: Quinolones (e.g., ciprofloxacin), or TMP-SMX, or Macrolides (e.g., clarithromycin or azithromycin) for 14-21 days. Patients with underlying cardiac valvular defects: Doxycycline plus hydroxychloroquine 200 mg PO tid for 12 months

Chronic Q Fever: Doxycycline plus quinolones for 4 years, or doxycycline plus hydroxychloroquine for 1.5-3 years.

COMMENTS

DoD Q-Fever vaccine manufactured in 1970. Significant side effects if administered inappropriately; sterile abscesses if prior exposure/skin testing required before vaccination. Time to develop immunity – 5 weeks.

Initiation of postexposure prophylaxis within 7 days of exposure merely delays incubation period of disease.

Tetracyclines are preferred antibiotic for treatment of acute Q fever except in

1. Meningoencephalitis: fluoroquinolones may penetrate CSF better than tetracyclines
2. Children < 8 yrs (doxycycline relatively contraindicated): TMP/SMX or macrolides (especially clarithromycin or azithromycin).
3. Pregnancy: TMP/SMX 160 mg/800 mg PO bid for duration of pregnancy. If evidence of continued disease at parturition, use tetracycline or quinolone for 2-3 weeks. Doxycycline is contraindicated during pregnancy.

(A) Approved for this use by the FDA
(IND) Available as an investigational new drug for this indication (i.e., NOT an FDA-approved use)

TULAREMIA

VACCINE/TOXOID

Live attenuated vaccine (USAMRIID-LVS, Preexposure) (IND) DoD Laboratory Use Protocol for vaccine. Single 0.1 ml dose via scarification in at-risk researchers.

Dynport Vaccine Company (DVC-LVS) undergoing Phase II trial for safety and immunogenicity in comparison with USAMRIID-LVS

CHEMOPROPHYLAXIS

Ciprofloxacin: 500 mg PO q 12 h for 14 d, 20mg/kg (up to 500 mg) PO bid (peds), **or**

Doxycycline: 100 mg PO bid x 14 d (adults), 2.2mg/kg (up to 100 mg) PO bid (peds<45 kg), **or**

Tetracycline: 500 mg PO qid x 14 d (adults)

CHEMOTHERAPY

Streptomycin: 1 g IM q12 h days x at least 10 days (adults)[A], 15mg/kg (up to 2g/day) IM q12h (peds) [A], or

Gentamicin: 5 mg/kg IM or IV qd, or 2 mg/kg loading dose followed by 1.7 mg/kg IM or IV q 8 h x at least 10 days (adults), 2.5 mg/kg IM or IV q 8 h (peds), **or**

Alternatives:

Ciprofloxacin 400 mg IV q 12 h for at least 10d (adults), 15 mg/kg (up to 400 mg) IV q 12 h (peds), **or**

Doxycycline: 200 mg IV, then 100 mg IV q 12 h x 14-21 d (adults)[A], 2.2 mg/kg (up to 100 mg) IV q 12 h (peds<45 kg), **or**

Chloramphenicol: 25 mg/kg IV q 6 h x 14-21 d, **or**

Tetracycline: 500 mg PO qid x 14-21 d (adults)[A]

COMMENTS

Vaccine manufactured in 1964.

Streptomycin is not widely available in the US and therefore is of limited utility. Gentamicin, although not approved for treatment of tularemia likely represents a suitable alternative. Adjust gentamicin dose for renal failure

Treatment with streptomycin, gentamicin, or ciprofloxacin should be continued for 10 days; doxycycline and chloramphenicol are associated with high relapse rates with course shorter than 14-21 days. IM or IV doxycycline, ciprofloxacin, or chloramphenicol can be switched to oral antibiotic to complete course when patient clinically improved.

Chloramphenicol is contraindicated in children less than 2 years. While chloramphenicol is potentially an alternative for postexposure prophylaxis (25 mg/kg PO qid), oral formulations are available only outside the US.

BOTULINUM NEUROTOXIN

VACCINE/TOXOID

Pentavalent (ABCDE) Toxoid (IND) Vaccine (Preexposure use only). IND for preexposure prophylaxis for high risk individuals (i.e., laboratorians) only. (IND)

Recombinant Botulinum Toxin Vaccine A/B (rBV A/B). IND for preexposure prophylaxis for high-risk individuals only. (IND)

CHEMOPROPHYLAXIS

DoD equine antitoxins(IND)

In general, botulinum antitoxin is not used prophylactically. Under special circumstances, if the evidence of exposure is clear in a group of individuals, some of whom have well defined neurological findings consistent with botulism, treatment can be contemplated in those without neurological signs.

CHEMOTHERAPY

Heptavalent (A-G) equine botulinum antitoxin (H-BAT) (Cangene Corporation) available through the CDC. IND for postexposure prophylaxis. (IND)

BabyBig™, California Health Department, types A and B Human lyophilized IgG, for treatment of infant botulism(A)

HE-BAT, DoD heptavalent despeciated equine botulism antitoxin, types A-G (IND)

HFabBAT, DoD de-speciated heptavalent equine botulism antitoxin, types A-G (IND))

COMMENTS

Decline in immunogenicity of the Pentavalent Toxoid Vaccine – current lot PBP-003 passed potency testing only to Serotypes A and B.

May need to perform skin test for hypersensitivity before equine antitoxin administration. Antitoxin levels observed 2-4 weeks after dose 3 of the primary series (week 13).

(A) Approved for this use by the FDA
(IND) Available as an investigational new drug for this indication (i.e. NOT an FDA-approved use)

RICIN TOXIN

VACCINE/TOXOID

Genetically modified toxin subunit vaccine (RiVax) undergoing Phase 1 clinical trials at USAMRIID. No licensed FDA vaccine available.

CHEMOPROPHYLAXIS

None

CHEMOTHERAPY

None

COMMENTS

Inhalation: supportive therapy.

G-I: gastric lavage, cathartics.

STAPHYLOCOCCUS ENTEROTOXINS

VACCINE/TOXOID

Inhibitex, Inc, and Pfizer have partnered to develop a three-antigen *S. aureus* vaccine (SA3Ag), and have completed Phase 1 trials. No licensed FDA vaccine available.

CHEMOPROPHYLAXIS

None

CHEMOTHERAPY

None

COMMENTS

Inhalation: supportive therapy.

G-I: gastric lavage, cathartics.

ENCEPHALITIS VIRUSES

VACCINE/TOXOID

JE inactivated vaccine JE-VAX[R] (Sanofi-Pasteur) [(A)] JE inactivated vaccine JE-VC (Ixiaro), does not contain thimerosal [(A)]

VEE Live Attenuated Vaccine[(IND)] (DoD Laboratory Use Protocol for Preexposure)

TC-83 strain

VEE Inactivated Vaccine[(IND)] (DoD Laboratory Use Protocol for Preexposure)

C-84 strain, given only for declining titers after receiving TC-83 vaccine or as a primary vaccination series for those failing to have a titer after receiving TC-83 vaccine

EEE Inactivated Vaccine[(IND)] (DoD Laboratory Use Protocol for Preexposure)

WEE Inactivated Vaccine[(IND)] (DoD Laboratory Use Protocol for Preexposure)

CHEMOPROPHYLAXIS

None

CHEMOTHERAPY

No specific therapy. Treatment consists of corticosteroids, anticonvulsants, and supportive care measures.

COMMENTS

Adverse events for alphavirus vaccines ~50%

VEE TC-83 vaccine manufactured in 1965. Live attenuated vaccine, with significant side effects. About 25% of vaccine recipients experience clinical reactions requiring bed rest. No seroconversion in 20%. Only effective against subtypes 1A, 1B, and 1C. VEE C-84 vaccine used for non-responders to TC-83. Preexisting immunity to a live *Alphavirus* vaccine inhibits vaccination with a second, different *Alphavirus* vaccine.

EEE and WEE vaccines are poorly immunogenic. Multiple boosters are required:

EEE vaccine manufactured in 1989. Antibody response is poor. Requires three-dose primary (1 month apart) and 1-2 boosters (1 month apart). Time to develop immunity – 3 months.

WEE vaccine manufactured in 1991. Antibody response is poor. Requires three-dose primary (1 month apart) and 3-4 boosters (1 month apart). Time to develop immunity – 6 months.

(A) Approved for this use by the FDA

(IND) Available as an investigational new drug for this indication (i.e., NOT an FDA-approved use)

HEMORRHAGIC FEVER VIRUSES

VACCINE/TOXOID

Yellow fever live attenuated 17D vaccine, given as a single shot, with a booster dose every 10 years. [A]

AHF vaccine [IND] (Cross-protection for BHF)

MP-12 attenuated RVF vaccine[IND] (DoD IND for high-risk laboratory workers)

TBE vaccine approved in Europe. Hantavirus vaccine approved in the Republic of Korea.

CHEMOPROPHYLAXIS

Lassa fever and CCHF: Ribavirin optimal dose and duration unknown, not FDA approved for this use.

CHEMOTHERAPY

Ribavirin for confirmed or suspected arenavirus, bunyavirus, or VHF of unknown etiology:

Loading dose (adults): 30 mg/kg IV (max 2 g) once; 2000 mg PO once

Maintenance dose (adults): 16 mg/kg IV (max 1 gram) q6 h for 4 days, 8 mg/kg IV (max 500 mg) q8 h for 6 days;

Wt > 75 kg: 600 mg PO bid for 10 days, Wt < 75 kg: 400 mg PO in AM, 600 mg PO in PM for 10 days

Loading dose (peds): IV same as for adult. 30 mg/kg PO once.

Maintenance dose (peds): IV same as for adult. 7.5 mg/kg PO bid for 10 days

Ribavirin (CCHF/Lassa) [IND] :

Loading Dose: 33 mg/kg (max dose: 2.64g), followed by

Day 1-4: 16 mg/kg (max dose: 1.28 g) q6 hours

Day 5-10: 8mg/kg (max dose: 0.64 g) q8hrs

COMMENTS

Aggressive supportive care and management of hypotension and coagulopathy very important.

Human antibody used with apparent beneficial effect in uncontrolled human trials of AHF.

Human experience with postexposure oral ribavirin use is anecdotal following exposures to CCHF and Lassa. Any use for this purpose should be under IND.

Consensus statement in JAMA from 2002 (see Table 2. *Recommended ribavirin dosing for treatment of viral hemorrhagic fevers,* in the Viral Hemorrhagic Fevers (VHF) chapter) suggests using ribavirin to treat clinically apparent hemorrhagic fever virus infection of unknown etiology using doses from CCHF/Lassa/HFRS IND.

SMALLPOX

VACCINE/TOXOID

Cell culture-derived vaccines (all NYCBOH strain):

- Dynport Vaccine (Preexposure)[(IND)]
- Acambis Vaccine (ACAM2000) (Preexposure)[(A)]

CHEMOPROPHYLAXIS

- Acambis Vaccine (ACAM2000) (Postexposure)[(A)]

CHEMOTHERAPY

Cidofovir for treatment of smallpox or severe or unexpected adverse event following smallpox vaccination[(IND)]:

- Probenecid 2g PO 3 hours before cidofovir infusion.
- infuse 1L NS 1 hours before cidofovir infusion
- Cidofovir 5 mg/kg IV over 1 hour
- repeat probenecid 1g PO 2 h and again 8 hours after cidofovir infusion completed.

For Select Vaccine Adverse reactions (Eczema vaccinatum, vaccinia necrosum, ocular vaccinia w/o keratitis, severe generalized vaccinia):

1. VIGIV (Vaccinia Immune Globulin, Intravenous). (Cangene Corporation) 6000U/kg IV infusion. 9000 U/kg for the patient that does not respond to the 6000 U/kg dose. See CDC guidelines at www.bt.cdc.gov/agent/smallpox/vaccination/mgmt-adv-reactions.asp

   VIG is NOT recommended for mild instances of accidental implantation, implantation-associated ocular keratitis, mild or limited generalized vaccinia, erythema multiforme, or encephalitis postvaccination)
2. Cidofovir 5 mg/kg IV infusion (as above)[(IND)]
3. ST-246 (oral dosage) [(IND)]

COMMENTS

Pre- and postexposure vaccination recommended if > 3 years since last vaccine.

Recommendations for use of smallpox vaccine in response to bioterrorism are periodically updated by the Centers for Disease Control and Prevention (CDC), and the most recent recommendations can be found at http:www.cdc.gov.

(A) Approved for this use by the FDA
(IND) Available as an investigational new drug for this indication (i.e,. NOT an FDA-approved use)

APPENDIX E: MEDICAL SAMPLE COLLECTION FOR BIOAGENTS

This guide helps determine which clinical samples to collect from individuals exposed to aerosolized biological threat agents or environmental samples from suspect sites. Proper collection of specimens from patients is dependent on the time-frame after exposure. Sample collection is described for "Early post-exposure," "Clinical," and "Convalescent/ Terminal/ Postmortem" time-frames. These time-frames are not rigid and will vary according to the concentration of the agent used, the agent strain, and predisposing health factors of the patient.

- Early postexposure: when it is known that an individual has been exposed to a bioagent aerosol; aggressively attempt to obtain samples as indicated
- Clinical: samples from those individuals presenting with clinical symptoms
- Convalescent/Terminal/Postmortem: samples taken during convalescence, the terminal stages of infection or toxicosis or postmortem during autopsy

Shipping Samples: Most specimens sent rapidly (less than 24 hours) to analytical labs require only blue or wet ice or refrigeration at 2 to 8°C. However, if the time span increases beyond 24 hours, contact the USAMRIID "Hot-Line" (1-888-USA-RIID) for other shipping requirements such as shipment on dry-ice or in liquid nitrogen.

Blood samples: Several choices are offered based on availability of the blood collection tubes. Do not send blood in all the tubes listed, but merely choose one. Tiger-top tubes that have been centrifuged are preferred over red-top clot tubes with serum removed from the clot, but the latter will suffice. Blood culture bottles are also preferred over citrated blood for bacterial cultures.

Pathology samples: Routinely include liver, lung, spleen, and regional or mesenteric lymph nodes. Additional samples requested are as follows: brain tissue for encephalomyelitis cases (mortality is rare), adrenal gland for Ebola (nice to have but not absolutely required) and bone marrow.

Culture of bone marrow for brucellosis has higher sensitivity than blood culture (Gotuzzo, et al.).

Fixatives: While 10% buffered formalin is the standard pathology fixative, it will prevent any cell culture. This is important, as infections are frequently not bacteremic or only intermittently bacteremic. If the transit time is short and/or refrigerated, samples can be sent in sterile normal saline. Formalin is an excellent tissue penetrator, but it interferes with polymerase chain reaction (PCR) and reverse transcriptase - polymerase chain reaction (RT-PCR) testing by degrading sample RNA and DNA. Alcohols also produce excellent tissue histology, although pathologists are not used to testing samples immersed in alcohol. Alcohols have low tissue penetration, so tissue samples should be sliced thin (3-4 mm) or minced for fixation. The volume of any fixative (formalin, alcohol etc.) should be several times the volume of tissue.

The gold standard for storage of PCR samples is -70°c or in liquid nitrogen; obviously liquid nitrogen may not be readily available outside of fixed facilities. There are also specialized products available: Ambion's RNAlader is a tissue preservative for RNA at room temperature. Biomatrica (www.biomatrica.com) has a full range of products for room temperature storage of samples for molecular testing. Specialized products may not be necessary, however, especially in a field-expedient situation. DNA and RNA viruses are detectable by PCR/RT-PCR even after 6 months of room temperature storage in alcohol. This was demonstrated in 100% ethanol, but would probably work in other alcohols. (Reid et al.)

The world has changed since the WHO Smallpox Eradication Program routinely shipped and carried thousands of live smallpox samples without creating any concern or incidents as was normal for all diagnostic and research samples. It was said at that time that samples were carried "VIP" (Virus in Pocket). Since then, a confusing maze of laws and regulations from multiple authorities that control shipment of biological samples has occurred since the 2001 anthrax mailings. Although written for a study of insect vector samples, Coleman et al. provides an excellent summary, which is excerpted below. Confusion and ambiguity has made many scientists reluctant to go on record with useful shipping advice. For example, the fact sheets and internet resources referenced by Coleman in September 2009 were quickly withdrawn. It is exceedingly difficult to obtain reliable shipping advice for biological pathogens. This effect of this confusion is to impede research, put patients at medical risk, and medical personnel at legal risk. Laboratories and shippers are afraid to act, precious samples thaw at borders, etc. The American Type Culture Collection, formerly the definite reference collection in microbiology, simply disposed of their extensive collection of select agents.

With this in mind, there appears to be three basic approaches available to people left with the responsibility to do practical work: 1. Send the samples as general diagnostic samples without testing or with only preliminary testing (or presumably definitive diagnosis of the patient from which they came.) 2. Fix or otherwise kill the samples rendering them suitable only for PCR, serology, or staining methods, but not culture or further characterization. 3. Ship samples which have been definitely identified as select agents with the arduous required safe guards and permits. Utilization of couriers on military aircraft or the medical evacuation chain may facilitate the process, though it of course doesn't obviate regulatory requirements.

"The U.S. Code of Federal Regulations (CFR) Title 49 is the document that governs the transportation of hazardous materials, to include infectious substances. ... [Samples are] considered general diagnostic specimens unless a specific pathogen has been identified or is suspected. Regulations pertaining to the air shipment of general diagnostic specimens include 9 CFR (Animal and Plant Health Inspection Service), 21 CFR (Food and Drug Administration), and 42 CFR (Centers for Disease Control and Prevention). To ensure that proper protection is in place to contain any undetected pathogenic micro-organisms, general diagnostic specimens should be packaged in accordance with International Air Transportation Association (IATA) Dangerous Goods regulations. In general, procedures for packing general diagnostic specimens for air shipment include (i) sample placed in a primary watertight receptacle with a leakproof seal, (ii) watertight receptacle wrapped in absorbent material, (iii) wrapped container placed in a secondary watertight receptacle, (iv) the entire package is placed in a strong outer packaging approved by the U.S, Department of Transportation (DOT) for transport of the hazardous material, (v) itemized list describing contents placed in the unsealed shipping box and (vi) designated certifying official approves package for transport. If needed, ice, dry ice, or pre-frozen packs should be placed between the secondary watertight receptacle and the outer packaging. Packages containing dry ice must permit the release of carbon dioxide. Diagnostic samples in which an infectious agent has been detected are no longer considered general diagnostic samples but rather are considered infectious substances. Infectious substances are defined as "a viable micro-organism, or its toxin, that causes or may cause disease in humans or animals, and includes those agents listed in 42 CFR 72.3 of the regulations of the Department of Health and Human Services or any other agent that causes or may cause severe, disabling or fatal disease."

"Very stringent regulations pertain to the shipment of infectious substances, with requirements described in detail in 49 CFR Part 173,196, The shipment of infectious substances requires coordinated action by the shipper, the transporter, and the receiver to ensure safe transport and arrival on time. Based on the definition of infectious substances as a "viable micro-organism," diagnostic samples containing a pathogen inactivated using appropriate grinding medium or diluent are considered general diagnostic samples and not infectious substances. As such, the less stringent procedures pertaining to the shipment of general diagnostic samples apply. Depending on the type of samples (e.g.. dead arthropods, general diagnostic sample, or infectious substances), appropriate CDC or U.S, Department of Agriculture (USDA) permits may be required to ship samples to the United States, biological select agents and toxins. Certain microbial pathogens and toxins that potentially pose a severe threat to human, animal, or plant health are referred to as biological select agents and toxins (BSATs). The U.S. Department of Health and Human Services and the USDA have regulatory authority over BSAT that can affect human and animal/plant health, respectively..... Laws regulating BSATs include Section 511 of the antiterrorism and Effective Death Penalty Act of 1996, the Uniting and Strengthening America by Providing Appropriate Tools Required to Intercept and Obstruct Terrorism Act of 2001 (USA PATRIOT Act), and the Public Health Security and Bioterrorism Preparedness and Response Act of 2002 (Bioterrorism Act), On March 18. 2005, HHS and USDA published the final Select Agent Regulations (42 CFR Part 73, 7 CFR Part 331. 9 CFR Part 121) in the Federal Register."

"Subsequent to the publication of these regulations, the DoD and each of the military services have published specific instructions pertaining to BSATs. to include DoD Instructions 5210.88 (Safeguarding Biological .Select Agents and Toxins) and 5210.89 (Minimum Security Standards for

Safeguarding Biological Select Agents and Toxins), Army Regulations 50-1 (Biological Surety), and 190-17 (Biological Select Agent and Toxins Security Program), and Air Force Policy Directive 10-39 (Safeguarding Biological Select Agents and Toxins). A number of BSATs are transmitted by arthropods, to include African swine fever, bluetongue, CCHF, EEE, JE, RVF, TBE, and VEE viruses, as well as *Rickettsia prowazekii*, *R. rickettsii*, *Franciscella tularensis*, and *Yersinia pestis*. Each of these pathogens could potentially be detected in arthropods during military deployments. Because of the severe threat posed by BSATs, the handling, transport, security, destruction, and reporting of these agents are highly regulated."

While the various regulations provide clear guidance on procedures used within the United States, there is little guidance on the detection and identification of BSATs in vectors during military deployments. Accepted practice during military deployments is to implement procedures that best meet the intent of relevant U.S, BSAT laws and regulations. A key issue during military deployments is to determine whether a diagnostic sample should be considered a BSAT, as determination that a sample is a BSAT triggers a variety of specific actions/responses. In general, diagnostic samples are only considered to contain BSATs once a viable pathogen has been identified using a confirmatory assay (42 CFR 73). As described previously, a true confirmatory assay should consist of two separate, validated tests that detect different targets on different genes. There are currently no field-deployable vector assays that meet this requirement; therefore, vector samples are normally considered "presumptive positives" and would not be considered BSATs. However, the future development and fielding of true confirmatory assays could potentially result in vector samples being classified as BSAT."

"An additional issue is the fact that procedures used to prepare samples for both screening and confirmatory diagnostic assays frequently inactivate any pathogens that are present, so that even though a confirmatory assay identified a particular pathogen, that sample would not be considered BSAT as no viable pathogen is present. However, laboratory personnel should use caution when making a determination that a positive sample is not a BSAT as it is extremely difficult in a field setting to determine whether a viable pathogen is present. Additionally, any portion of the diagnostic sample that did not undergo nucleic acid extraction or other sterilizing procedures that would have inactivated the infectious virus may still contain viable BSATs (if identified by a confirmatory assay) and should be destroyed within 7 days as specified in 42 CFR 73. To further complicate matters, nucleic acid from positive-stranded RNA viruses can be used to produce infectious virus—this material would be considered a BSAT, if detected using a confirmatory assay. Clearly, personnel conducting diagnostic testing for BSATs should understand the rules and regulations pertaining to BSATs. Criteria for determining if a sample contains a BSAT should be established, as should procedures for securing, transporting, and destroying these samples per Army, DoD, and U.S. laws and regulations. Personnel conducting diagnostic testing must also understand that samples that do not meet the strict definition of a BSAT may still pose a considerable threat to anyone exposed to these samples. For example, a sample that tests positive for RVF virus using a hand-held screening assay is not considered a BSAT; however, a potentially lethal virus may still be present in the sample if the grinding diluent does not completely inactivate the pathogen."

BACTERIA AND RICKETTSIA

Early post-exposure	Clinical	Convalescent/ Terminal/Postmortem
Anthrax Bacillus anthracis <u>0 – 24 h</u> Nasal and throat swabs, induced respiratory secretions for culture, FA, and PCR	<u>24 to 72 h</u> Serum (TT, RT) for toxin assays Blood (E, C, H) for PCR. Blood (BC, C) for culture	<u>3 to 10 days</u> Serum (TT, RT) for toxin assays Blood (BC, C) for culture. Pathology samples
Plague Yersinia pestis <u>0 – 24 h</u> Nasal swabs, sputum, induced respiratory secretions for culture, FA, and PCR	<u>24 – 72 h</u> Blood (BC, C) and bloody sputum for culture and FA (C), F-1 Antigen assays (TT, RT), PCR (E, C, H)	<u>>6 days</u> Serum (TT, RT) for IgM later for IgG. Pathology samples
Tularemia Francisella tularensis <u>0 – 24 h</u> Nasal swabs, sputum, induced respiratory secretions for culture, FA and PCR	<u>24 – 72 h</u> Blood (BC, C) for culture Blood (E, C, H) for PCR Sputum for FA & PCR	<u>>6 days</u> Serum (TT, RT) for IgM and later IgG, agglutination titers. Pathology Samples
BC: Blood culture bottle C: Citrated blood (3-ml)	E: EDTA (3-ml) H: Heparin (3-ml)	TT: Tiger-top (5 – 10 ml) RT: Red top if no TT

BACTERIA AND RICKETTSIA

Early post-exposure	Clinical	Convalescent/ Terminal/Postmortem
Glanders Burkholderia mallei <u>0 – 24 h</u> Nasal swabs, sputum, induced respiratory secretions for culture and PCR.	<u>24 – 72 h</u> Blood (BC, C) for culture Blood (E, C, H) for PCR Sputum & drainage from skin lesions for PCR & culture.	<u>>6 days</u> Blood (BC, C) and tissues for culture. Serum (TT, RT) for immunoassays. Pathology samples.
Brucellosis Brucella abortus, suis, & melitensis <u>0 – 24 h</u> Nasal swabs, sputum, induced respiratory secretions for culture and PCR.	<u>24 – 72 h</u> Blood (BC, C) for culture. Blood (E, C, H) for PCR.	<u>>6 days</u> Blood (BC, C) and tissues for culture. Serum (TT, RT) for immunoassays. Pathology samples
Q-Fever *Coxiella burnetii* <u>0 – 24 h</u> Nasal swabs, sputum, induced respiratory secretions for culture and PCR.	<u>2 to 5 days</u> Blood (BC, C) for culture in eggs or mouse inoculation Blood (E, C, H) for PCR.	<u>>6 days</u> Blood (BC, C) for culture in eggs or mouse inoculation Pathology samples.
BC: Blood culture bottle C: Citrated blood (3-ml)	E: EDTA (3-ml) H: Heparin (3-ml)	TT: Tiger-top (5 – 10 ml) RT: Red top if no TT

TOXINS

Early post-exposure	Clinical	Convalescent/ Terminal/Postmortem
Botulism Botulinum toxin from Clostridium botulinum		
0 – 24 h Nasal swabs, induced respiratory secretions for PCR (contaminating bacterial DNA) and toxin assays. Serum (TT, RT) for toxin assays	24 to 72 h Nasal swabs, respiratory secretions for PCR (contaminating bacterial DNA) and toxin assays.	>6 days Usually no IgM or IgG Pathology samples (liver and spleen for toxin detection)
Ricin Intoxication Ricin toxin from castor beans		
0 – 24 h Nasal swabs, induced respiratory secretions for PCR (contaminating castor bean DNA) and toxin assays. Serum (TT) for toxin assays	36 to 48 h Serum (TT, RT) for toxin assay Tissues for immunohistological stain in pathology samples.	>6 days Serum (TT, RT) for IgM and IgG in survivors
Staph enterotoxicosis Staphylococcus Enterotoxin B		
0 – 3 h Nasal swabs, induced respiratory secretions for PCR (contaminating bacterial DNA) and toxin assays. Serum (TT, RT) for toxin assays	2 - 6 h Urine for immunoassays Nasal swabs, induced respiratory secretions for PCR (contaminating bacterial DNA) and toxin assays. Serum (TT, RT) for toxin assays	>6 days Serum for IgM and IgG Note: Only paired antibody samples will be of value for IgG assays…most adults have antibodies to staph enterotoxins.
T-2 toxicosis		
0 – 24 h postexposure Nasal & throat swabs, induced respiratory secretions for immunoassays, HPLC/ mass spectrometry (HPLC/MS).	1 to 5 days Serum (TT, RT), tissue for toxin detection	>6 days postexposure Urine for detection of toxin metabolites
______	______	______
______	______	______
BC: Blood culture bottle	E: EDTA (3-ml)	TT: Tiger-top (5 – 10 ml)
C: Citrated blood (3-ml)	H: Heparin (3-ml)	RT: Red top if no TT

VIRUSES

Early post-exposure	Clinical	Convalescent/ Terminal/Postmortem
Equine Encephalomyelitis VEE, EEE and WEE viruses 0 – 24 h Nasal swabs & induced respiratory secretions for RT-PCR and viral culture (in viral transport medium)	24 to 72 h Serum & Throat swabs for culture (TT, RT), RT-PCR (E, C, H, TT, RT) and Antigen ELISA (TT, RT), CSF, Throat swabs up to 5 days	>6 days Serum (TT, RT) for IgM Pathology samples plus brain
Ebola 0 – 24 h Nasal swabs & induced respiratory secretions for RT-PCR and viral culture (in viral transport medium)	2 to 5 days Serum (TT, RT) for viral culture	>6 days Serum (TT, RT) for viral culture. Pathology samples plus adrenal gland.
Pox (Smallpox, monkeypox) *Orthopoxvirus* 0 – 24 h Nasal swabs & induced respiratory secretions for PCR and viral culture (in viral transport medium)	2 to 5 days Serum (TT, RT) for viral culture	>6 days Serum (TT, RT) for viral culture. Drainage from skin lesions/ scrapings for microscopy, EM, viral culture, PCR. Pathology samples
BC: Blood culture bottle C: Citrated blood (3-ml)	E: EDTA (3-ml) H: Heparin (3-ml)	TT: Tiger-top (5 – 10 ml) RT: Red top if no TT

Environmental samples can be collected to determine the nature of a bioaerosol either during, shortly after, or considerably after an attack. Obviously, the sooner that the environmental sample is taken, in conjunction with early postexposure clinical samples, can help to identify the agent in time to initiate prophylactic treatment.

Samples taken well after an attack may allow identification of the agent used. While this information would likely be too late for useful prophylactic treatment, when combined with other information, may be used in the prosecution of war crimes or other criminal proceedings. Although not strictly a medical responsibility, sample collection concerns are the same as for during or shortly after a bioaerosol attack, and medical personnel may be the only personnel with the requisite training.

If time and conditions permit, medical postexposure planning and risk assessments should be performed. As in any hazmat situation, a clean line and exit and entry strategy should be designed. Depending on the situation, personnel protective equipment should be donned. The standard M40 gas mask is effective protection against bioaerosols. If it is possible to have a clean line, then a three-person team is recommended, with one clean and two dirty. The former would help decontaminate the latter. The samples may be used in a criminal prosecution, what, where, when, how, etc of the sample collection should be documented both in writing and with pictures. Consider using waterproof disposable cameras, and waterproof notepads Because these items may need to be decontaminated. The types of samples taken can be extremely variable. Some of the possible samples are:

- Aerosol collections in buffer solutions
- Soil
- Swabs
- Dry powders
- Container of unknown substance
- Vegetation
- Food / water
- Body fluids or tissues

What is collected will depend on the situation. Aerosol collection during an attack would be ideal, assuming you have the appropriate collection device. Otherwise anything that appears to be contaminated can be either sampled with swabs if available, or with absorbent paper or cloth. The item itself could be collected if not too large. Well after the attack, samples from dead animals or human remains can be taken (refer to Appendix F for appropriate specimens). All samples should ideally be double bagged in Ziploc bags (the outside of the inner bag decontaminated with dilute bleach before placing in the second bag) labeled with time and place of collection along with any other pertinent data.

APPENDIX F: SPECIMENS FOR LABORATORY DIAGNOSIS

Disease	Face or Nasal Swab[1]	Blood Culture	Smear	Acute & Convales-cent Sera	Stool	Urine	Other
Anthrax	+	+	Pleural & CS fluids mediastinal lymph node spleen	+	+/–	–	Cutaneous lesion aspirates or 4mm punch biopsy, toxin detection
Brucellosis	+	+	–	+	–	–	Bone marrow and spinal fluid cultures; tissues, exudates
Cholera	–	–	–	+	+	–	
Glanders & Melioidosis	+	+	Sputum and abscess aspirates	+	–	+/–	Abscess culture
Plague	+	+	Sputum	+	–	–	Bubo aspirate, CSF, sputum, lesion scraping, lymph node aspirate
Tularemia	+	+	+[2]	+	–	–	
Q-fever	+	+[4]	Lesions	+	–	–	Lung, spleen, lymph nodes, bone marrow biopsies
Venezuelan Equine Encephalitis	+	[3]	–	+	–	–	CSF
Viral Hemor-rhagic Fevers	+	[3]	–	+	–	–	Liver
Botulism	+	–	–	+	–	–	Serum or other fluids for toxin detection/ mouse bioassay
Staph Enterotoxin B	+	–	–	+	+	+	Lung, kidney
Ricin Toxin	+	–	–	+	+	+	Spleen, lung, kidney
T-2 Mycotoxins	+	–	–	–	+	+	Serum, stool, or urine for metabolites
Clostridial Toxins	+	–	Wound tissues	+	+	–	

[1]Within 18-24 hr of exposure

[2]Fluorescent antibody test on infected lymph node smears. Gram stain has little value

[3]Virus isolation from blood or throat swabs in appropriate containment

[4]*C burnetii* can persist for days in blood and resists desiccation. EDTA anticoagulated blood preferred. Culturing should not be done except in biosafety level-3 containment

APPENDIX G: BIOAGENT LABORATORY IDENTIFICATION

				Immunoassays			
Disease	Agent	Gold Standard	Antigen Detection	IgG	IgM	PCR	Animal
Aflatoxin	Aflatoxins	Mass spectrometry	X				
Anthrax	Bacillus anthracis	FA/Std Microbiology	X	X	X	X	X
Brucellosis	Brucella sp	FA/Std Microbiology	X	X	X	X	X
Cholera	Vibrio cholerae	Std Microbiology/ serology	X(toxin)	X	X	X	
Glanders	B mallei	Std Microbiology		X	X	X	
	B pseudomallei	Std Microbiology		X	X	X	
Plague	Yersinia pestis	FA/Std Microbiology	X	X	X	X	X
Tularemia	F tularensis	FA/Std Microbiology	X	X	X	X	X
Q Fever	*C burnetii*	FA/eggs or cell Cx/serology	X	X	X	X	X
Smallpox	Orthopox Viruses	Virus isolation/ FA/ neutralization	X	X		X	X
Venezuelan Equine Encephalitis	Arboviruses (incl. alphaviruses)	Virus isolation/FA, neutralization	X	X	X	X	X
Viral Hemorrhagic Fevers	Filoviruses	Virus isolation/ neutralization	X	X	X	X	X
	Hantaviruses	Virus isolation/ FA/ neutralization	X	X	X	X	X
Botulism	Bot Toxins (A-G)/C botulinum	Mouse neutraliza- tion/ standard microbiology	X			*	X
Saxitoxin	Saxitoxin	Bioassay		(neutralizing antibodies)		X	
Shigellosis	Shigella sp	Std Microbiology	X			X	
Staph Enterotoxin B	SEB Toxin	ELISA	X	X		*	X
Ricin	Ricin Toxin	ELISA	X	X	X	X	X
T-2 Mycotoxins	T-2 Mycotoxins	Mass spectrometry	X				
Tetrodototoxin	Tetrodotoxins	Bioassay	X	(neutralizing antibodies)			X
	C. perfringens/ toxins	Std. Micro./ELISA (alpha & enterotoxin)	X	X		X	

*Toxin gene detected – only works if cellular debris including genes present as contaminant. Purified toxin does not contain detectable genes.

ELISA - enzyme-linked immunosorbent assays

FA - indirect or direct immunofluorescence assays

Std Micro/serology - standard microbiological techniques available, including electron microscopy

Not all assays are available in field laboratories

APPENDIX H: DIFFERENTIAL DIAGNOSIS OF CHEMICAL NERVE AGENT, BOTULINUM TOXIN AND SEB INTOXICATION FOLLOWING INHALATION EXPOSURE

	Chemical Nerve Agent	Botulinum Toxin	SEB
Time to Symptoms	Minutes	Hours (12-48)	Hours (1-6)
Nervous	Convulsions, Muscle twitching	Progressive, descending skeletal muscle flaccid paralysis	Headache, Muscle aches
Cardiovascular	Slow heart rate	Normal rate	Normal or rapid heart rate
Respiratory	Difficult breathing, airway constriction	Normal, then progressive paralysis	Nonproductive cough; Severe cases; chest pain/difficult breathing
Gastrointestinal	Increased motility, pain, diarrhea	Decreased motility	Nausea, vomiting and/or diarrhea
Ocular	Small pupils	Droopy eyelids, Large pupils, disconjugate gaze	May see "red eyes" (conjunctival infection)
Salivary	Profuse, watery saliva	Normal; difficulty swallowing	May be slightly increased quantities of saliva
Death	Minutes	2-3 days	Unlikely
Response to Atropine/ 2PAM-CL	Yes	No	Atropine may reduce gastrointestinal symptoms

APPENDIX I: COMPARATIVE LETHALITY OF SELECTED TOXINS & CHEMICAL AGENTS IN LABORATORY MICE[1]

Agent	LD_{50} (µg/kg)	Molecular Weight	Source
Botulinum neurotoxin A	0.001	150,000	Bacterium
Shiga toxin	0.002	55,000	Bacterium
Tetanus toxin	0.002	150,000	Bacterium
Abrin	0.04	65,000	Plant (Rosary Pea)
Diphtheria toxin	0.10	62,000	Bacterium
Maitotoxin	0.10	3,400	Marine Dinoflagellate
Palytoxin	0.15	2,700	Marine Soft Coral
Ciguatoxin	0.40	1,000	Marine Dinoflagellate
Textilotoxin	0.60	80,000	Elapid Snake
C. perfringens toxins	0.1– 5.0	35-40,000	Bacterium
Batrachotoxin	2.0	539	Arrow-Poison Frog
Ricin (Aerosol)	3.0	64,000	Plant (Castor Bean)
alpha-Conotoxin	5.0	1,500	Cone Snail
Taipoxin	5.0	46,000	Elapid Snake
Tetrodotoxin	8.0	319	Puffer Fish
alpha-Tityustoxin	9.0	8,000	Scorpion
Saxitoxin	10.0 (Inhal 2.0)	299	Marine Dinoflagellate
VX	15.0	267	Chemical Agent
SEB (rhesus/aerosol)	27.0 (ED_{50}~pg)	28,494	Bacterium
Anatoxin-a(S)	50.0	500	Blue-Green Algae
Microcystin	50.0	994	Blue-Green Algae
Soman (GD)	64.0	182	Chemical Agent
Sarin (GB)	100.0	140	Chemical Agent
Aconitine	100.0	647	Plant (Monkshood)
T-2 Toxin	1,210.0	466	Fungal Myotoxin

[1]Unless otherwise stated, LD_{50} data is determined by intravenous route, and marine toxins are determined by intraperitoneal route

APPENDIX J: AEROSOL TOXICITY IN LD_{50} VS. QUANTITY OF TOXIN

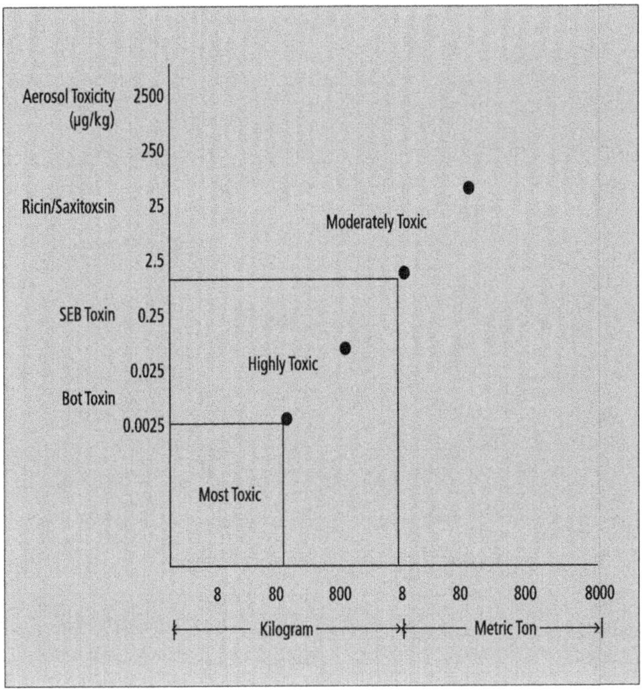

Aerosol toxicity in LD_{50} (see Appendix C) vs quantity of toxin required to provide a theoretically effective open-air exposure, under ideal meteorological conditions, to an area 100 km.[2] Ricin, saxitoxin, and botulinum toxins kill at the concentrations depicted (Patrick and Spertzel, 1992: Based on Cader KL, BWL Tech Study #3, Mathematical models for dosage and casualty resulting from single point and line source release of aerosol near ground level, DTIC#AD3 10-361, Dec 1957).

APPENDIX K: REFERENCES

Introduction / History of Biological Warfare and the Current Threat

1. Alibek K Biohazard Random House, New York 1999
2. Carus WS Bioterrorism and Biocrimes: The Illicit Use of Biological Agents Since 1900 National Defense University, Center for Counterproliferation Research, Fredonia Books, 2002
3. CDC Investigation of a ricin-containing envelope at a postal facility--South Carolina, 2003 MMWR 52:1129-31 2003
4. Christopher GW, Cieslak TJ, Pavlin JA, Eitzen EM Biological warfare A historical perspective JAMA 278:412-7 1997
5. Fenn E Pox Americana Hill & Wang, 2002
6. Geissler E, Ellis van Courtland Moon J, eds Biological and Toxin Weapons: Research, Development and Use from the Middle Ages to 1945 Stockholm International Peace Research Institute Oxford University Press 1999
7. Harris SH Factories of Death New York, NY Routledge, 1994
8. Mayor A Greek Fire, Poison Arrows & Scorpion Bombs: Biological and Chemical Warfare in the Ancient World The Overlook Press, New York, 2003
9. McIsaac, JH Preparing Hospitals for Bioterror: A Medical and Biomedical Systems Approach Academic Press/Elsevier, Burlington, MA 2006
10. Meselson M, Guillemin J, Hugh-Jones M, Langmuir A, et al The Sverdlovsk anthrax outbreak of 1979 Science 266:1202-8 1994
11. Noah DL, Huebner KD, Darling RG, Waeckerle J, The history and threat of biological warfare and terrorism Emerg Med Clin North Am 20:255-71 2002
10 Speirs EM A History of Chemical and Biological Weapons Reaktion Books, London, UK 2010
11 Takahashi H, Keim P, Kaufmann AF, Keys C, Sm,ith K, Taniguchi K, Inouye S, Kurata T *Bacillus anthracis* bioterrorism Incident, Kameido, Tokyo, 1993 Emerg Infect Dis 10:117-20 2004
12 Torok TJ, Tauxe RV, Wise RP, Livengood JR, Sokolow R, Mauvais S, Birkness KA, Skeels MR, Horan JM, Foster LR A large community outbreak of salmonellosis caused by intentional contamination of restaurant salad bars JAMA 278:389-95 1997

Distinguishing Between Natural and Intentional Disease Outbreaks

1. Ashford DA, Kaiser RM, Bales ME, Shutt K, Patrawalla A, McShan A, Tappero JW, Perkins BA, Dannenberg AL Planning against biological terrorism: lessons from outbreak investigations Emerg Infect Dis 9:515-9 2003
2. Breeze RG, Budowle B, Schutzer SE, eds Microbial Forensics Elsevier Academic Press, Burlington, MA 2005
3. Dembek ZF, Kortepeter MG, Pavlin, JA Discernment between deliberate and natural infectious disease outbreaks Epidemiol Infect 137:353-371 2007
4. Dembek ZF, Buckman RL, Fowler SK, Hadler JL Missed sentinel case of naturally occurring pneumonic tularemia outbreak: lessons for detection of bioterrorism J Am Board Fam Pract 16:339-42 2003
5. Franz DR, Jahrling PB, Friedlander AM, McClain DJ, Hoover DL, Bryne WR, Pavlin JA, Christopher GW, Eitzen EM Jr Clinical recognition and management of patients exposed to biological warfare agents JAMA 278:399-411 1997
6. Grunow R, Finke EJ A procedure for differentiating between the intentional release of biological warfare agents and natural outbreaks of disease: its use in analyzing the tularemia outbreak in Kosovo in 1999 and 2000 Clin Microbiol Infect 8:510-21 2002

7. Hugh-Jones M Distinguishing between natural and unnatural outbreaks of animal diseases Rev Sci Tech 25:173-186 2006
8. Keim P, Smith KL, Keys C, Takahashi H, Kurata T, Kauffman A Molecular investigation of the Aum Shinrikyo anthrax release in Kameido, Japan J Clin Microbiol 39:4566-4567 2001
9. Noah DL, Sobel AL, Ostroff SM, Kildew JA Biological warfare training: infectious disease outbreak differentiation criteria Mil Med 163:198-201 1998
10. Pavlin J Epidemiology of bioterrorism Emerg Infect Dis 5:528-30 1999
11. Reintjes R, Dedushaj I, Gjini A, Jorgensen TR, Cotter B, Lieftucht A, D'Ancona F, Dennis DT, Kosoy MA, Mulliqi-Osmani G, Grunow R, Kalaveshi A, Gashi L, Humolli I Tularemia outbreak investigation in Kosovo: case control and environmental studies Emerg Infect Dis 8:69-73 2002
12. Reissman DB, Steinberg EB, Magri JM, Jernigan DB The anthrax epidemiologic tool kit: an instrument for public health preparedness Biosecur Bioterror 1:111-6 2003
13. Takahashi H, Keim P, Kaufmann AF, Keys C, Smith KL, Taniguchi K, Inouye S, Kurata T *Bacillus anthracis* incident, Kameido, Tokyo, 1993 Emerg Infect Dis 10:117-20 2004 Errata - Emerg Infect Dis 10:385 2004
14. Treadwell TA, Koo D, Kuker K, Khan AS Epidemiologic clues to bioterrorism Public Health Rep Mar-Apr;118(2):92-8 2003
15. Zelicoff AP An Epidemiological Analysis of the 1971 Smallpox outbreak in Aralsk, Kazakhstan Crit Rev Microbiol 29:97-108 2003

Medical Management

1. Binder P, Attre O, Boutin JP, Cavallo JD, Debord T, Jouan A, Vidal D Medical management of biological warfare and bioterrorism: place of the immunoprevention and the immunotherapy Comp Immunol Microbiol Infect Dis 26:401-421 2003
2. Cieslak TJ, Rowe JR, Kortepeter MG, Madsen JM, Newmark J, Christopher GW, Culpepper RC, Eitzen EM A field-expedient algorithmic approach to the clinical management of chemical and biological casualties Mil Med 165:659-62 2000
3. Cieslak TJ Henretig FM Medical consequences of biological warfare: the ten commandments of management Mil Med 166[suppl 2]:11-12 2001
4. Cone DC, Koenig KL Mass casualty triage in the chemical, biological, radiological, or nuclear environment Eur J Emerg Med 6:287-302 2005
5. Franz DR, Jahrling PB, Friedlander AM, McClain DJ, Hoover DL, Byrne WR, Pavlin JA, Christopher GW, Eitzen EM Clinical recognition and management of patients exposed to biological warfare agents JAMA 278:399-411 1997
6. Henretig FM, Cieslak TJ, Kortepeter MG, Fleisher GR Medical management of the suspected victim of bioterrorism: an algorithmic approach to the undifferentiated patient Emerg Med Clin North Am 20:351-64 2002
7. Rusnak JM, Kortepeter MG, Aldis J, Boudreau E Experience in the medical management of potential laboratory exposures to agents of bioterrorism on the basis of risk assessment at the United States Army Medical research Institute of Infectious Diseases (USAMRIID) J Occupational Environ Med 46:801-811 2004
8. White SR, Henretig FM, Dukes RG Medical management of vulnerable populations and co-morbid conditions of victims of bioterrorism Emerg Med Clin North Am 20:365-392 2002

Anthrax

1. Chitlaru T, Altboum Z, Reuveny S, Shafferman A Progress and novel strategies in vaccine development and treatment of anthrax Immunol Rev 239:221-236 2011
2. Cieslak TJ, Eitzen EE Jr Clinical and Epidemiologic Principles of Anthrax Emerg Infect Dis 5:552-5 1999
3. Cybulski RJ Jr, Sanz P, O'Brien AD Anthrax vaccination strategies Mol Aspects Med 30:490-502 2009

4. Dewan PK, Fry AM, Laserson K, Tierney BC, Quinn CP, Hayslett JA, Broyles LN, Shane A, Winthrop KL, Walks I, Siegel L, Hales T, Semenova VA, Romero-Steiner S, Elie C, Khabbaz R, Khan AS, Hajjeh RA, Scuchat A, and members of the Washington, DC, Anthrax Response Team Inhalational anthrax outbreak among postal workers, Washington, DC, 2001 Emerg Infect Dis 8:1066-72 2002
5. Dupuy LC, Schmaljohn CS DNA vaccines for biodefense Expert Rev Vaccines 8:1739-1754 2009
6. Fasanella A, Galante D, Garafolo D, Jones MH Anthrax undervalued zoonosis Vet Microbiol 140:318-331 2010
7. Fennelly KP, Davidow AL, Miller SL, Connell N, Ellner J Airborne infection with *Bacillus anthracis*—from mills to mail Emerg Infect Dis 10:996-1001 2004
8. Friedlander AM, Little SF Advances in the development of next-generation anthrax vaccines Vaccine 27(Suppl 4):D28-32 2009
9. Inglesby TV, Henderson DA, John G Bartlett JG, and colleagues; for the Working Group on Civilian Biodefense Anthrax as a biological weapon JAMA 281;1735-1745 1999
10. Inglesby TV, O'Toole T, MD, MPH; Henderson, DA; for the Working Group on Civilian Biodefense Anthrax as a biological weapon, 2002: updated recommendations for management JAMA 287:2236-2252 2002
11. Klinman DM, Yamamoto M, Tross D, Tomaru K Anthrax prevention and treatment: utility of therapy combining antibiotic plus vaccine Expert Opin Biol Ther 9:1477-1486 2009
12. CDC Use of anthrax vaccine in the United States: Recommendations of the Advisory Committee on Immunization Practices (ACIP), 2009 MMWR 59 (RR-6):1-30 2010
13. Vietri NJ, Purcell BK, Tobery SA, Rasmussen SL, Leffel EK, Twenhafel NA, Ivins BE, Kellogg WM, Wright ME, Friedlander AM A very short course in antibiotic treatment is effective in preventing death from experimental inhalational anthrax after discontinuing antibiotics J Infect Dis 199:336-341 2009
14. Vietri NJ, Purcell BK, Lawler LJ, Leffel EK, Rico P, Gamble CS, Twenhafel NA, Ivins BE, Heine HS, Sheeler R, Wright ME, Friedlander AM Short-course postexposure antibiotic prophylaxis combined with vaccination protects against experimental inhalational anthrax Proc Natl Acad Sci 103:7813-7816 2006

Brucellosis

1. CDC Brucellosis outbreak at a pork processing plant -- North Carolina, 1992 MMWR 43:113-116 1994
2. Colmenero JD, Reguera JM, Martos F, et alComplications associated with Brucella melitensis infection: a study of 530 cases Medicine 75:195-211 1996
3. Harris NL, McNeely WF, Shepard J-A O, et al Weekly clinicopathological exercises: case 22-2002 N Engl J Med 347:200-206 2002
4. Lopez-Goni I, Moriyon I Brucella: Molecular and Cellular Biology Horizon Bioscience, Wyndmonhan, UK 2004McLean DR, Russell N, Khan MY, 1992
5. McLean DR, Russell N, Khan MY Neurobrucellosis: clinical and therapeutic features Clin Infect Dis 15:582-590 1992
6. Nielsen K, Duncan JR, eds Animal Brucellosis CRC Press, LLC Boca Raton, FL 1990Neubauer H Brucellosis: New demands in a changing world Prilozi 31:209-217 2010
7. Solera J, Martinez-Alfaro E, and Espinosa A Recognition and optimum treatment of brucellosis Drugs 53:245-256 1997
8. CDC Suspected brucellosis case prompts investigation of possible bioterrorism-related activity - New Hampshire and Massachusetts, 1999 MMWR 49:509-512 2000
9. Teske SS, Huang Y, Tamraker SB, Bartrand TA, Weir MH, Haas CN Animal and human dose-response models for Brucella species Risk Anal 2011 Mar 30 doi: 101111/j1539-6924201101602x [Epub ahead of print]
10. Young EJ, Corbel MJ, eds Brucellosis: clinical and laboratory aspects CRC Press, LLC Boca Raton, FL 1989

Glanders / Melioidosis

1. Bondi SK, Goldberg JB Strategies towards vaccines against *Burkholderia pseudomallei* and *Burkholderia mallei* Expert Rev Vaccines 7:1357-1365 2009
2. CDC Laboratory-acquired human glanders - Maryland, May 2000 MMWR 49(24);532-5 2000
3. Cheng AC, Currie BJ Melioidosis: Epidemiology, pathophysiology, and management Crit Microbiol Rev 18:383-416 2005
4. Cheng AC, Fisher DA, Anstey NM, Stephens DP, Jacups SP, Currie BJ Outcomes of patients with melioidosis treated with meropenem Antimicrob Agents Chemother 48:1763-5 2004
5. Coenye T, Vandamme P, eds Burkholderia: Molecular Microbiology and Genomics Horizon Bioscience, Wyndmondham, UK 2006
6. Howe C, Miller WR Human glanders: report of six cases Ann Intern Med1:93-115 1947
7. Kosuwon W, Taimglang T, Sirichativapee W, Jeeravipoolvarn P Melioidotic septic arthritis and its risk factors J Bone Joint Surg Am 85-A:1058-61 2003
8. Larsen JC, Johnson NH Pathogenesis of *Burkholderia pseudomallei* and *Burkhoderia mallei* Mil Med 174:647-651 2009
9. Neubauer, H, Meyer, H, Finke, EJ Human glanders Revue Internationale Des Services De Sante Des Forces Armees 70:258-265 1997
10. O'Brien M, Freeman K, Lum G, Cheng AC, Jacups SP, Currie BJ Further evaluation of a rapid diagnostic test for melioidosis in an area of endemicity J Clin Microbiol 42:2239-40 2004
11. Russell P, Eley SM, Ellis J, Green M, Bell DL, Kenny DJ, Titball RW Comparison of efficacy of ciprofloxacin and doxycycline against experimental melioidosis and glanders J Antimicrob Chemother 45:813-818 2000
12. Srinivasan A, Kraus CN, DeShazer D, Becker PM, Dick JD, Spacek L, Bartlet JG, Byrne WR, Thomas DL Glanders in a military research microbiologist N Engl J Med 4:256-258 2001
13. Steele JH: Glanders In: Steele JH (ed) CRC Handbook Series in Zoonoses, Section A: Bacterial, Rickettsial and Mycotic Diseases, Vol I CRC Press, Boca Raton, FL, pp 339-362 1979
14. Verma RD Glanders in India with special reference to incidence and epidemiology Indian Vet J 58:177-183 1981
15. Warawa J, Woods DE Melioidosis vaccines Expert Rev Vaccines 1:477-82 2002
16. Wittig MB, Wohlsein P, Hagen RM, Al Dahouk S, Tomaso H, Scholtz HC, Nikolaou K, Wernery R Glanders – a comprehensive review Dtsch Tierarztl Wochenschr (German) 113:323-330 2006

Plague

1. Boulanger LL, Ettestad P, Fogarty JD, Dennis DT, Romig D, Mertz G Gentamicin and tetracyclines for the treatment of human plague: review of 75 cases in New Mexico, 1985-1999 Clin Infect Dis 38:663-9 2004
2. Butler T Plague into the 21st century Clin Infect Dis 49:736-742 2009
3. Campbell GL, Dennis DT Plague and other *Yersinia* infections In: Kasper DL, et al; eds Harrison's Principles of Internal Medicine 14th ed McGraw Hill, NY, NY pp975-83 1998
4. Centers for Disease Control and Prevention Prevention of plague Recommendations of the Advisory Committee on Immunization Practices (ACIP) MMWR 45(RR-14):1-151996
5. Dennis DT and Gage JL Plague In: Armstrong D and Cohen J (eds) Infectious Diseases London: Mosby, Armstrong, and Cohen, 1999
6. Dennis, DT, Gage KL, Gratz N, Poland JD, and Tikhomirov E Plague manual: epidemiology, distribution, surveillance and control Geneva: World Health Organization 1999 171 pp WHO/CDS/CSR/EDC/992
7. Fritz CL, Dennis DT, Tipple MA, Campbell GL, McCance CR, and Gubler DJ Surveillance for pneumonic plague in the United States during an international emergency: a model for control of imported emerging diseases Emerg Infect Dis 2:30-361996

8. Gage KL Plague In: Colliers L, Balows A, Sussman M, Hausles WJ, eds Topley and Wilson's Microbiology and Microbiological Infections, vol 3 London: Edward Arnold Press pp885-9031998
9. Gage KL, Kosoy MY Natural history of plague: perspectives from more than a century of research Annu Rev Entomol 50:505-528 2005
10. Inglesby TV, Dennis DT, Henderson DA, Bartlett JG, et al Plague as a biological weapon: medical and public health management JAMA 283:2281-90 2000
11. Perry RD, Fetherston JD *Yersinia pestis* -- etiologic agent of plague Clin Microbiol Rev 10:35-66 1997
12. Poland JD, Barnes AM Plague In Steele J (ed): Handbook of Zoonoses CRC Press , Boca Raton, FL pp515-559 1979
13. Smiley ST Immune defense against pneumonic plague Immunol Rev 225:256-271 2008
14. Stenseth NC, Atshabar BB, Begon M, Belmain SR, Bertherat E, Carniel E, Gage KL, Leirs H, Rahalison L Plague: Past present, and future PLoS Med 5(1):1e 2008 Jan 15
15. Teh W-L Treatise on Pneumonic Plague League of Nations Original Report 466 pp 1926

Q Fever

1. Anderson AD, Baker TR, Littrell AC, Mott RL, Niebuhr DW, Smoak BL Seroepidemiologic survey for *Coxiella burnetii* among hospitalized US troops deployed to Iraq Zoonoses Publ Health 58:276-283 2011
2. Burnet FM, Freeman M Experimental studies on the virus of "Q" fever Med J Australia 1:299-305 1937
3. Fenollar F, Fournier P, Carrieri M, Habib G, Messana T and Raoult D Risks factors and prevention of Q fever endocarditis Clin Infect Dis 33:312-6 2001
4. Gefenaite G, Munster JM, van Houdt R, Hak E Effectiveness of the Q fever vaccine: A meta-analysis Vaccine 29:395-298 2011
5. Gikas A, Kokkini S, Tsioutis C Q fever: Clinical manifestations and treatment Expert Rev Anti Infect Ther 8:529-539 2010
6. Levy PY, Drancourt M, Etienne J, Auvergnat JC, Beytout J, Sainty JM, Goldstein F, Raoult D Comparison of different antibiotic regimens for therapy of 32 cases of Q fever endocarditis Antimicrob Agents Chemother 35:533-7 1991
7. Marrie TJ *Coxiella burnetti* (Q fever) pneumonia Clin Infect Dis 21(Suppl 3):S253-S264 1995
8. Marrie TJ, ed Q fever, Volume I: The disease CRC Press, LLC Boca Raton, FL 1990
9. Maurin M, Raoult D Q fever Clin Microbiol Rev 12:518-53 1999
10. Q Fever - California, Georgia, Pennsylvania, and Tennessee, 2000—2001 MMWR 51:924-927 2002
11. Raoult D, Fenollar F and Stein A Q fever during pregnancy: diagnosis, treatment, and follow-up Arch Intern Med162:701-4 2002
12. Raoult D Treatment of Q fever Antimicrob Agents Chemother 37: 1733-6 1993
13. Sampere M, Font B, Font J, et al Q fever in adults: review of 66 clinical cases Eur J Clin Microbiol Infect Dis 22:108-110 2003
14. Williams JC, Thompson HA, eds Q fever, Volume II: The biology of *Coxiella burnetii* CRC Press Boca Raton, FL 1991

Tularemia

1. CDC Tularemia—United States, 1990-2000 MMWR 8;51(9):182-184 2002
2. CDC Tularemia --- Missouri, 2000-2007 MMWR 58:744-748 2009
3. Dembek ZF, Buckman RL, Fowler SK, Hadler JH Missed sentinel case of naturally occcurring pneumonic tularemia outbreak: lessons for detection of bioterrorism J Am Board Fam Prac 16:339-342 2003
4. Dennis DT, Inglesby TV, Henderson DA, Bartlett JG, et al Tularemia as a biological weapon: medical and public health management JAMA 285:2763-73 2001

5. Evans ME, Gregory DW, Schaffner W, McGee ZA Tularemia: A 30-year experience with 88 cases Medicine (Baltimore) 64:251-269 1985

6. Feldman KA, Enscore RE, Lathrop SL, Matyas BT, McGuill BT, Scriefer ME, Stikles-Enos D Dennis DT, Peterson LR, Hayes EB An outbreak of primary pneumonic tularemia on Martha's Vineyard N Eng J Med 345:1601-1606 2001

7. Feldman KA, Stiles-Enos D, Julian K, Matyas BT, Telford SR 3rd, Chu MC, Peterson LR, Hayes EB Tularemia on Martha's Vineyard: seroprevalence and occupational risk Emerg Infect Dis 9:350-354 2003

8. Foshay L Effects of serum treatment in 600 cases of acute tularemia JAMA 110:603 1938

9. Francis E Tularemia JAMA 84:1243-1250 1925

10. Grunow R A procedure for differentiating between the intentional release of biological warfare agents and natural outbreaks of disease: its use in analyzing the tularemia outbreak in Kosovo in 1999 and 2000 Clin Microbiol Infect 8:510-21 2002

11. Reintjes R, Dedushaj I, Gjini A, Rikke-Jorgensen T, Cotter B, Lieftucht A, D'Ancona F, Dennis DT, Kosoy MA, Mulliqi-Osmani G, Grunow R, Kalaveshi A, Gashi L, and Humolli I Tularemia outbreak investigation in Kosovo: case control and environmental studies Emerg Infect Dis 8:69-73 2002

12. Siderowski SH, ed Tularemia Infobase Publishing, NY, NY 2006

13. Simpson W Tularemia: History, Pathology, Diagnosis and Treatment Paul B Hoeber, Inc New York 1929

14. Snowden J, Stovall S Tularemia: Retrospective review of 10 years' experience in Arkansas Clin Pediatr (Phila) 50:64-68 2011

15. Teutsch SM, Martone WJ, Brink EW, Potter ME, Eliot G, Hoxsie R, Craven RB, Kauffman AF Pneumonic tularemia on Martha's Vineyard New Engl J Med 1979; 301:826-828 1979

16. Thomas LD, Schaffner W Tularemia pneumonia Infect Dis Clin North Am 24:43-55 2010

Smallpox

1. Bray M, Buller M Looking back at smallpox Clin Infect Dis 38:882-9 2004

2. Breman JG, Henderson DA Diagnosis and management of smallpox N Engl J Med 346:1300-8 2002

3. CDC Secondary and tertiary transfer of vaccinia virus Among US military personnel - United States and worldwide, 2002-2004 MMWR 53:103-105 2004

4. CDC Smallpox vaccination and adverse reactions 52(RR04):1-28 2003

5. CDC Recommendations for using smallpox vaccine in a pre-event vaccination program MMWR 52(RR07)1-16 2003

6. CDC Vaccinia virus infection after sexual contact with a military smallpox vaccine – Washington, 2010 MMWR 59:773-775 2010

7. Redfield RR, Wright DC, James WD, Jones TS, Brown C, Burke DS Disseminated vaccinia in a military recruit with human immunodeficiency virus (HIV) disease N Engl J Med 316:673-6 1987

8. Fenner F, Henderson DA, Arita I, Jezek Z, Ladnyi ID Smallpox and its eradication WHO 1460 pp 1988

9. Henderson DA, Inglesby TV, Bartlett JG, et al Smallpox as a biological weapon Medical and public health management JAMA 281:2127-2137 1999

10. CDC Human monkeypox-Kasai Oriental, Democratic Republic of Congo (Zaire), 1996-1997 MMWR 46:301-71 1997

11. Kesson A, Ferguson JK, Rawlinson WD, Cunningham AL Progressive vaccinia treated with ribavirin and vacinia immune globulin Clin Infect Dis 25:911-4 1997

12. McClain DJ, Harrison S, Yeager CL, et al Immunologic responses to vaccinia vaccines administered by different parenteral routes J Infect Dis 175:756-63 1997

13. CDC Vaccinia (Smallpox) vaccine: recommendations of the ACIP MMWR, 40:RR-14 (Suppl) 1991

Venezuelan Equine Encephalitis

1. Bowen GS, Calisher CH Virological and serological studies of Venezuelan equine encephalomyelitis in humans J Clin Microbiol 4:22-7 1976
2. Bowen GS, Fashinell TR, Dean PB, Gregg MB Clinical aspects of human Venezuelan equine encephalitis in Texas Bull Pan Am Health Organ 10:46-57 1976
3. de la Monte S, Castro F, Bonilla NJ, Gaskin de Urdaneta A, Hutchins GM The systemic pathology of Venezuelan equine encephalitis virus infection in humans Am J Trop Med Hyg 34:194-202 1985
4. Durbin AP, Whitehead SS Dengue vaccine candidates in development Curr Top Microbiol Immunol 338:129-143 2010
5. Paessler S, Weaver SC Vaccines for Venezuelan equine encephalitis Vaccine 27(Suppl 4):D80-D85 2009
6. Reed DS, Lind CM, Sullivan LJ, Pratt WD, Parker MD Aerosol infection of cynomolgus macaques with enzootic strains of Venezuelan equine encephalitis viruses J Infect Dis 189:1013-7 2004
7. Reichert E, Clase A, Bacetty A, Laersen J Alphavirus antiviral drug development: scientific gap analysis and prospective research areas Biosecur Bioterror 7:413-427 2009
8. Rivas F, Diaz LA, Cardenas VM, et al Epidemic Venezuelan equine encephalitis in La Guajira, Colombia, 1995 J Infect Dis 175:828-32 1997
9. Steele KE, Twenhafel NA Pathology of animal models of alphavirus encephalitis Vet Pathol 47:790-805 2010
10. Watts DM, Callahan J, Rossi C, et al Venezuelan equine encephalitis febrile cases among humans in the Peruvian Amazon River region Am J Trop Med Hyg 58:35-40 1998
11. Weaver SC, Ferro C, Barrera R, Boshell J, Navarro JC Venezuelan equine encephalitis Annu Rev Entomol 49:141-74 2004
12. Zacks MA, Paessler S Encephalitic alphaviruses Vet Microbiol 140:281-286 2010

Viral Hemorrhagic Fevers

1. Armstrong LR, Dembry LM, Rainey PM, Russi MB, Khan AS, Fischer SH, Edberg SC, Ksiazek TG, Rollin PE, Peters CJ Management of a Sabia virus-infected patient in a US Hospital Infect Control Hosp Epidemiol 20:176-82 1999
2. Auguste AJ, Volk SM, Arrigo NC, Martinez R, Ramkissoon V, Adams AP, Thompson NN, Adesiyun AA, Chadee DD, Foster JE, Travassos Da Rosa APA, Tesh RB, Weaver SC, Carrington CVF Isolation and phylogenetic analysis of Mucambo virus (Venezuelan equine encephalitis complex subtype IIIA) in Trinidad Virology 392: 123-30 2009
3. Barry M, Russi M, Armstrong L, Geller D, Tesh R, Dembry L, Gonzalez JP, Khan AS, Peters CJ Brief report: treatment of a laboratory acquired Sabia virus infection N Engl J Med 333:294-6 1995
4. Borio L, Inglesby T, Peters CJ, Schmaljohn AL, Hughes JM, Jahrling PB, Ksiazek T, Johnson KM, Meyerhoff A, O'Toole T, Ascher MS, Bartlett J, Breman JG, Eitzen EM Jr, Hamburg M, Hauer J, Henderson DA, Johnson RT, Kwik G, Layton M, Lillibridge S, Nabel GJ, Osterholm MT, Perl TM, Russell P, Tonat K; Working Group on Civilian Biodefense Hemorrhagic fever viruses as biological weapons: medical and public health management JAMA 287(18):2391-405 2002
5. CDC Update: Filovirus infections among persons with occupational exposure to nonhuman primates MMWR 39:266-7 1990
6. CDC Update: Management of patients with suspected viral hemorrhagic fever-United States MMWR 44:475-9 1995
7. Christopher GW, Eitzen EM Jr Air evacuation under high-level biosafety containment: the aeromedical isolation team Emerg Infect Dis 241-246 1999

8. Fisher-Hoch SP, Price ME, Craven RB, et al Safe intensive-care management of a severe case of Lassa fever with simple barrier nursing techniques Lancet 2:1227-1229 1985
9. Holmes GP, McCormick JB, Trock SC, et al Lassa fever in the United States: investigation of a case and new guidelines for management N Engl J Med 323:1120-1123 1990
10. Jahrling PB, Geisbert TW, Dalgard DW, et al Preliminary report: isolation of Ebola virus from monkeys imported to USA Lancet 335:502-505 1990
11. Lukaszewski RA, Brooks TJ Pegylated alpha interferon is an effective treatment for virulent Venezuelan equine encephalitis virus and has profound effects on the host immune response to infection J Virol 74:5006-15 2000
12. Peters CJ, LeDuc JW, Breman JG, Jahrling PB, Rodier G, Rollin, PE, van der Groen, G Ebola: The virus and the disease J Infect Dis 179 Supplement 1 1999
13. Peters CJ, Sanchez A, Rollin PE, Ksiazek TG, Murphy FA Filoviridae: Marburg and Ebola viruses Fields Virology (3d ed), Fields BN, Knipe DM, Howley PM, et al (eds) Lippincott-Raven, Philadelphia pp 1161-76 1996
14. Phillpotts RJ, Jones LD, Howard SC Monoclonal antibody protects mice against infection and disease when given either before or up to 24 h after airborne challenge with virulent Venezuelan equine encephalitis virus Vaccine 20:1497-504 2002
15. Phillpotts RJ Venezuelan equine encephalitis virus complex-specific monoclonal antibody provides broad protection, in murine models, against airborne challenge with viruses from serogroups I, II and III Virus Res 120:107-12 2006

Botulism

1. Angulo FJ, Getz J, Taylor JP, Hendricks KA, Hatheway CL, Barth SS, Solomon HM, Larson AE, Johnson EA, Nickey LN, Ries AA A large outbreak of botulism: the hazardous baked potato J Infect Dis 178: 172-7 1998
2. Arnon SS, Schecter R, Inglesby TV, Henderson DA, et al Botulism toxin as a biological weapon: medical and public health management JAMA 285:1059-70 2001
3. Arnon SS, Schechter R, Maslanka SE, Jewell NP, Hatheway CL Human botulism immune globulin for the treatment of infant botulism N Engl J Med 354:462—71 2006
4. CDC Investigational Heptavalent botulinum antitoxin (HBAT) to replace licensed botulinum antitoxin AB and investigational botulinum antitoxin E MMWR 59(10):299 2010
5. Dembek ZF, Smith LA and Rusnak JM Botulism: Its cause, effects, diagnosis, clinical and laboratory identification and treatment modalities Disaster Med Public Health Prep 1:122-134 2007
6. CDC Botulism in the United States 1899 – 1996 Handbook for epidemiologists, clinicians, and laboratory workers 42 pp 1998
7. Hakami RM, Ruthel G, Stahl AM, Bavari S Gaining ground:assays for therapeutics against botulinum neurotoxin Trends Microbiol 18:164-172 2010
8. Rusnak JM, Smith LA Botulinum neurotoxin vaccines: past history and recent developments Hum Vacc 5:794-805 2009
9. Shapiro RL, Hatheway C, Becher J, Swerdlow DL Botulism surveillance and emergency response: a public health strategy for a global challenge JAMA 278: 433-5 1997
10. Shapiro RL, Hatheway C, Swerdlow DL Botulism in the United States: A clinical and epidemiologic review Ann Intern Med 129:221-8 1998
11. Smith LA Botulism and vaccines for its prevention Vaccine 27(Suppl 4):D33-D39 2009
12. CDC Wound botulism - California, 1995 MMWR 44:200-202 1995

Ricin

1. Audi J, Belson M, Patel M, Schier J, Osterloh J Ricin poisoning: a comprehensive review JAMA 294:2342-2351 2005
2. Bigalke H, Rummel A Medical aspects of toxin weapons Toxicology 214:210-220 2005

3. CDC Investigation of a ricin-containing envelope at a postal facility --- South Carolina, 2003 MMWR 52:1129-1131 2003
4. Challoner KR, McCarron MM Castor bean intoxication Ann Emerg Med 19:159-65 1990
5. Griffiths GD, Phillips GJ, Holley J Inhalation toxicology of ricin preparations: animal models, prophylactic and therapeutic approaches to protection Inhal Toxicol 19:873-87 2007
6. Marsden CJ, Smith DC, Roberts LM, Lord JM Ricin: current understanding and prospects for an antiricin vaccine Expert Rev Vaccines 4:229-37 2005
7. Musshoff F, Madea B Ricin poisoning and forensic toxicology Drug Test Anal 1:184-191 2009
8. Olsnes S, Kozlov JV Ricin Toxicon 39:1723-8 2001
9. Spivak L, Hendrickson RG Ricin Crit Care Clin 21:815-24 2005

Staphylococcal Enterotoxin B

1. Coffman JD, Zhu J, Roach JM, Bavari S, Ulrich RG, Giardina SL Production and purification of a recombinant Staphylococcal enterotoxin B vaccine candidate expressed in *Escherichia coli* Protein Expr Purif 24:302-12 2002
2. Henghold WB 2nd Other biologic toxin bioweapons: ricin, staphylococcal enterotoxin B, and trichothecene mycotoxins Dermatol Clin 22(3):257-62 2004
3. Mantis NJ Vaccines against the category B toxins: Staphylococcal enterotoxin B, epsilon toxin and ricin Adv Drug Deliv Rev 57:1424-39 2005
4. Morissette, C, J Goulet, and G Lamoureux Rapid and sensitive sandwich enzyme-linked immunosorbent assay for detection of staphylococcal enterotoxin B in cheese Appl Environ Microbiol 57:836-842 1991
5. Nedelkov, D, A Rasooly, and R W Nelson Multitoxin biosensor-mass spectrometry analysis: a new approach for rapid, real-time, sensitive analysis of staphylococcal toxins in food Int J Food Microbiol 60:1-13 2000
6. Rusnak JM, Kortepeter M, Ulrich R, Poli M, Boudreau E Laboratory exposures to staphylococcal enterotoxin B Emerg Infect Dis10:1544-9 2004
7. Schotte, U, N Langfeldt, A H Peruski, and H Meyer Detection of staphylococcal enterotoxin B (SEB) by enzyme-linked immunosorbent assay and by a rapid hand-held assay Clin Lab 48:395-400 2002
8. Seprenyi G, Shibata T, Onody R, Kohsaka T In staphylococcus enterotoxin B (SEB)-stimulated human PBMC, the LAK activity of non-T cells might have a major role in the mechanism of glomerular endothelial cells' injury Immunobiology 197:44-54 1997

Trichothecene Mycotoxins

1. Atroshi F, Rizzo A, Westermarck T, Ali-Vehmas T Antioxidant nutrients and mycotoxins Toxicology 180:151-67 2002
2. Hamaki T, Kami M, Kishi A, Kusumi E, Kishi Y, Iwata H, Miyakoshi S, Ueyama J, Morinaga S, Taniguchi S, Ohara K, Muto Y Vesicles as initial skin manifestation of disseminated fusariosis after non-myeloablative stem cell transplantation Leuk Lymphoma 45:631-3 2004
3. Holstege CP, Bechtel LK, Reilly TH, Wispelwey BP, Dobmeier SG Unusual but potential agents of terrorists Emerg Med Clin North Am 25:549-66 2007
4. Katz R, Singer B Can an attribution assessment be made for Yellow Rain? Systematic reanalysis in a chemical-and-biological-weapons use investigation Politics Life Sci 26:24-42 2007
5. Li FQ, Luo XY, Yoshizawa T Mycotoxins (trichothecenes, zearalenone and fumonisins) in cereals associated with human red-mold intoxications stored since 1989 and 1991 in China Nat Toxins 7:93-7 1999
6. Luo Y, Yoshizawa T, Katayama T Comparative study on the natural occurrence of Fusarium mycotoxins (trichothecenes and zearalenone) in corn and wheat from high- and low-risk areas for human esophageal cancer in China Appl Environ Microbiol 56:3723-6 1990

7. Rosen RT, Rosen JD Presence of four *Fusarium* mycotoxins and synthetic material in 'yellow rain' Evidence for the use of chemical weapons in Laos Biomed Mass Spectrom 9:443-50 1982
8. Sahu SC, O'Donnell MW Jr, Wiesenfeld PL Comparative hepatotoxicity of deoxynivalenol in rat, mouse and human liver cells in culture J Appl Toxicol30:566-73 2010
9. Schollenberger M, Suchy S, Jara HT, Drochner W, Muller HM A survey of *Fusarium* toxins in cereal-based foods marketed in an area of southwest Germany Mycopathologia147:49-57 1999
10. Sudakin DL Trichothecenes in the environment: relevance to human health Toxicol Lett 20;143:97-107 2003

Emerging Infections and Future Biological Weapons

1. Addressing Emerging Infectious Disease Threats: A Prevention Strategy for the United States Atlanta, Georgia: US Public Health Service, 1994
2. Black, John L, Genome projects and gene therapy: gateways to next generation biological weapons Milit Med 168, 11:864-71 2003
3. Bridges CB, Harper SA, Fukuda K, et al Prevention and control of influenza Recommendations of the Advisory Committee on Immunization Practices (ACIP) MMWR Recom Rep 2003 52(RR-8): 1-34 2003 Erratum in: MMWR 52:526 2003
4. CDC Addressing Emerging Infectious Disease Threats: A Prevention Strategy for the United States Atlanta, Georgia: US Public Health Service, 1994
5. CDC Revised US surveillance case definition for severe acute respiratory syndrome (SARS) and update on SARS cases - United States and worldwide, December 2003 MMWR 52:1202-1206 2003
6. Cox NJ, Bender CA The molecular epidemiology of influenza viruses Seminar in Virology 6:359-370 1995
7. Daly MJ The emerging impact of genomics on the development of biological weapons Clin Lab Med 21(3):619-29 2001
8. Domaradskij IV, Orent LW Achievements of the Soviet biological weapons programme and implications for the future Rev Sci Tech25:153-61 2006
9. Kagan E Bioregulators as Instruments of Terror Clin Lab Med21(3):607-18 2001
10. Gamblin SJ, Haire LF, Russell RJ, Stevens DJ, Xiao B, Ha Y, Vasisht N, Steinhauer DA, Daniels RS, Elliot A, Wiley DC, Skehel JJ The structure and receptor-binding properties of the 1918 influenza hemagglutinin, Science 303:1838-1842 2004
11. Gurley ES, Montgomery JM, Hossain MJ, Bell M, Azad AK, Islam MR, Molla MAR, Carroll DS, Ksiazek TG, Rota PA, Lowe L, Comer JA, Rollin P, Czub M, Grolla A, Feldmann H, Luby SP, Woodward JL, Breiman RF Person-to-Person Transmission of Nipah virus in a Bangladeshi community Emerg Infect Dis 13:1031-1037 2007
12. Harper SA, Fukuda K, Cox NJ, et al Using live, attenuated influenza vaccine for prevention and control of influenza: supplemental recommendations of the Advisory Committee on Immunization Practices (ACIP) MMWR 52(RR-13): 1-8 2003
13. Playford EG, McCall B, Smith G, Slinko V, Allen G, Smith I, Moore F, Taylor C, Kung Y-S, Field H Human Hendra virus encephalitis associated with equine outbreak, Australia 2008 EID 16:219-223 2010
14. CDC Revised US surveillance case definition for severe acute respiratory syndrome (SARS) and update on SARS cases – United States and worldwide, December 2003 MMWR 52:1202-1206 2003
15. Schrag SJ, Brooks JT, Van Beneden C, Parashar UD, Griffin PM, Anderson LJ, Bellini WJ, Benson RF, Erdman DD, Klimov A, Ksiazek TG, Peret TCT, Talkington DF, Thacker WL, Tondella ML, Sampson JS, Hightower AW, Nordenberg DF, Plikaytis BD, Khan AS, Rosenstein NE, Treadwell TA, Whitney CG, Fiore, AE, Durant TM, Perz JF, Wasley A, Feikin D, Herndon JL, Bower WA, Kilbourn BW, Levy DA, Coronado VG, Buffington J, Dykewicz CA, Khabbaz RF 2004 SARS surveillance during emergency public health response, United States, March-July 2003 Emerg Infect Dis 10:185-194 2004

Detection

1. Ackelsberg J, Leykam FM, Hazi Y, Madsen LC, West TH, Faltesek A, Henderson GD, Henderson CL, Leighton T The NYC Native Air Sampling Pilot Project: Using HVAC filter data for urban biological incident characterization Biosecur Bioterror 2011 Jul 27

2. Begier EM, Barrett NL, Mshar PA, Johnson DG, Hadler JL; Connecticut bioterrorism field epidemiology response team Emerg Infect Dis 11:1483-1486 2005

3. Bravata DM, Sundaram V, McDonald KM, Smith WM, Szeto H, Schleinitz MD, Owens DK Evaluating detection and diagnostic decision support systems for bioterrorism response Emerg Infect Dis 10:100-108 2004

4. Espy MJ, Cockerill III FR, Meyer RF, Bowen MD, Poland GA, Hadfield TL, Smith TF Detection of smallpox virus DNA by LightCycler PCR J Clin Microbiol 40:1985-8 2002 Erratum in: J Clin Microbiol 40:4405 2002

5. Field PR, Mitchell JL, Santiago A, Dickeson DJ, Chan SW, Ho DW, Murphy AM, Cuzzubbo AJ, Devine PL Comparison of a commercial enzyme-linked immunosorbent assay with immunofluorescence and complement fixation tests for detection of *Coxiella burnetii* (Q fever) immunoglobulin M J Clin Microbiol 38:1645-7 2000

6. Johnasson A, Berglund L Erikkson U, Goransson I, Wollin R, Forsman M, Tarnvik A, Sjostedt A Comparative analysis of PCR versus culture for diagnosis of ulceroglandular tularemia J Clin Microbiol 38:22-6 2000

7. Kulesh DA, Baker RO, Loveless BM, Norwood D, Zwiers SH, Mucker E, Hartmann C, Herrera R, Miller D, Christensen D, Wasieloski LP, Huggins J, Jahrling PB Smallpox and pan-orthopox virus detection by real-time 3'-minor groove binder TaqMan assays on the Roche LightCycler and the Cepheid Smart Cycler platforms J Clin Microbiol 42:601-9 2004

8. Kraft AE, Kulesh DA Applying molecular biological techniques to detecting biological agents Clin Lab Med 21:631-60 2001

9. Ligler FS, Taitt CR, Shriver-Lake LC, Sapsford KE, Shubin Y, Golden JP Array biosensor for detection of toxins Anal Bioanal Chem 377:469-77 2003

10. Lim DV, Simpson JM, Kearns, EA, Kramer MF Current and developing technologies for monitoring agents of bioterrorism and biowarfare Clin Microbiol Rev 18:583-607 2005

11. Maragos CM Novel assays and sensor platforms for the detection of aflatoxins Adv Exp Med Biol 504:85-93 2002

12. Probert WS, Schrader KN, Khuong NY, Bystrom SL, Graves MH Real-time multiplex PCR assay for detection of *Brucella* spp, *B abortus*, and *B melitensis* J Clin Microbiol 42:1290-3 2004

13. Rantakokko-Jalava K, Viljanen MK Application of *Bacillus anthracis* PCR to simulated clinical samples Clin Microbiol Infect 10:1051-6 2003

14. Tomaso H, Reisinger EC, Al Dahouk S, Frangoulidis D, Rakin A, Landt O, Neubauer H Rapid detection of *Yersinia pestis* with multiplex real-time PCR assays using fluorescent hybridisation probes FEMS Immunol Med Microbiol 38:117-26 2003

15. Uhl JR, Bell CA, Sloan LM, Espy MJ, Smith TF, Rosenblatt JE, Cockerill FR Application of rapid-cycle real-time polymerase chain reaction for the detection of microbial pathogens: the Mayo-Roche Rapid Anthrax test Mayo Clin Proc 77:673-80 2002

16. Varma-Basil M, El-Hajj H, Marras SAE, Hazbon MH, Mann JM, Connell ND, Kramer FR, Alland D Molecular beacons for multiplex detection of four bacterial bioterrorism agents Clin Chem 50:1060-1062 2004

17. Weidmann M, Muhlberger E, Hufert FT Rapid detection protocol for filoviruses J Clin Virol 30:94-9 2004

Personal Protection

1. 29 CFR 1910120, 130, 132, 134 series, http://wwwoshagov/pls/oshaweb/owadispshow_document?p_table=STANDARDS&p_id=9696

2. Brinker A, Prior K, Schumacher J Personal protection during resuscitation of casualties contaminated with chemical or biological warfare agents – a survey of medical first responders Prehosp Disaster Med 24:525-528 2009
3. FM 8-284 Treatment of Biological Warfare Agent Casualties, 115 pp 17 July 2000
4. CDC Biological and chemical terrorism: strategic plan for preparedness and response; recommendations of the CDC Strategic Planning Workgroup MMWR 49 (No RR-4):1–14 2000
5. Charney W Handbook of Modern Hospital Safety 2nd Edition CRC Press, Boca Raton, FL 1226 pp 2009
6. JP 3-11 Joint Doctrine for Operations in Nuclear, Biological, and Chemical (NBC) Environments, 139 pp 11 July 2000
7. USACHPPM Technical Guide 275 Personal Protective Equipment Guide for Military Medical Treatment Facility Personnel Handling Casualties from Weapons of Mass Destruction and Terrorism Events 220 pp Aug 2003
8. Recommendations for the Selection and Use of Protective Clothing and Respirators against Biological Agents April 2009
http://wwwcdcgov/niosh/docs/2009-132/
9. OSHA Best Practices for Hospital-Based First Receivers of Victims from Mass Casualty Incidents Involving the Release of Hazardous Substances January 2005 http://wwwoshagov/dts/osta/bestpractices/html/hospital_firstreceivershtml
10. Lavoie J, Cloutier Y, Lara J, Marchand G Guide on respiratory protection against bioaerosols Recommendations on its selection and use Chemical Substances and Biological Agents IRST Technical Guide RG-501 Montreal, Quebec 40 pp July 2007

Decontamination

1. FM 3-115 Multiservice Tactics, Techniques, and Procedures for Chemical, Biological, Radiological, and Nuclear (CBRN) Decontamination
2. Best Practices and Guidelines for Mass Personnel Decontamination, Technical Support Working Group (TSWG), 1st Ed, June 2003
3. FM 8-284 Treatment of Biological Warfare Agent Casualties, 17 July 2000
4. Hawley RJ, Eitzen EM Biological weapons- a primer for microbiologists Ann Rev Microbiol 55:235-253 2001
5. CDC Biological and chemical terrorism: strategic plan for preparedness and response; recommendations of the CDC Strategic Planning Workgroup MMWR 49(No RR-4):1–14 2000
6. JP 3-11 Joint Doctrine for Operations in Nuclear, Biological, and Chemical (NBC) Environments, 11 July 2000
7. Lawson JR, Jarboe TL, Aid for Decontamination of Fire and Rescue Service Protective Clothing and Equipment After Chemical, Biological, and Radiological Exposures, NIST Special Publication 981, May 2002
8. Raber E, Carlsen TM, Folks KJ, Kirvel RD, Dnaiels JI, Bogen KT How clean is clean enough? Recent developments in response to threats posed by chemical and biological warfare agents Int J Environ Health Res 14:31-41 2007
9.Rogers JV, Sabourin CLK, Choi YW, Richter WR, Rudnicki DC, Riggs KB, Taylor ML, Chang J Decontamination assessment of *Bacillus anthracis*, *Bacillus subtilis*, and *Geobacillus stearothermohilus* spores on indoor surfaces using a hydrogen peroxide gas generator J Appl Microbiol 99:739-748 2005

Investigational New Drugs

1. Code of Federal Regulations, title 21 – Food and Drugs, Parts 11, 50, 54, 56, 58, 201, 312, 314, 316 http://wwwfdagov/cder/regulatory/applications/ind_page_1htm#Introduction

2. Cummings ML Informed consent and investigational new drug abuses in the US military Account Res 9:93-103 2002
3. Food and Drug Administration, HHS Current good manufacturing practice and investigational new drugs intended for use in clinical trials Final rule Fed Regist 73(136):40453-40463 2008
4. Holbein ME Understanding FDA regulatory requirements for investigational new drug applications for sponsor-investigators Investig Med 57:688-694 2009
5. Kuhlmann J The application of biomarkers in early clinical drug development to improve decision-making processes Ernst Schering Res Found Workshop 59:29-45 2007
6. Sarapa N Exploratory IND: a new regulatory strategy for early clinical drug development in the United States Ernst Schering Res Found Workshop 59:151-163 2007
7. Woonnacott K, Lavole D, Fiorentino R, McIntyre M, Huang Y, Hirschfeld S Investigational new drugs submitted to the Food and Drug Administration that are placed on clinical hold: the experience of the Office of Cellular, Tissue and Gene Therapy Cyotherapy 10:312-316 2008

Appendix E Medical Sample Collection for Biological Threat Agents

1. Gotuzzo E, Carrillo C, Guerra J, Llosa L An evaluation of diagnostic methods for brucellosis--the value of bone marrow culture J Infect Dis 1986 Jan;153(1):122-5
2. Krafft, AE; Russell, KL; Hawksworth, AW; McCall, S; Irvine, M; Daum, LT; Connoly, JL; Reid, AH; Gaydos, JC; and Taubenberger, JK Evaluation of PCR testing on ethanol-fixed nasal swab specimens as an augmented surveillance strategy for influenza and adenoviruses J Clin Microbiol 43(4):1768-1775, Apr 2005
3. Coleman RE, Hochberg LP Putnam JL, Swanson KL, Lee JS, McAvin JC, Chan AS, O'Guinn ML Ryan JR, Wirtz RA, Moulton JK, Dave K, Faulde MK Use of Vector Diagnostics During Military Deployments: Recent Experience in Iraq and Afghanistan Mil Med 174, 9:904, 2009
4. Preparing Hazardous Materials for Military Air Shipments Air Force Manual 24-204 (Interservice) TM 38-250 1 September 2009

APPENDIX L: INVESTIGATIONAL NEW DRUGS (IND) AND EMERGENCY USE AUTHORIZATIONS (EUA)

OVERVIEW

It is DoD policy that personnel will be provided, when operationally relevant, the best possible medical countermeasures to chemical, biological, radiological, and nuclear (CBRN) agents and effects, and other health threats.

The DoD Components are expected to administer or use medical products (i.e., drugs or biologics) approved, licensed, or cleared by the FDA for general commercial marketing, when available, to provide the needed medical countermeasure.

Drugs are chemical substances intended for use in the medical diagnosis, cure, treatment, or prevention of disease. Biologics are blood and blood products, vaccines, allergenics, cell and tissue-based products, and gene therapy products.

Unapproved medical products or approved medical products used "off-label" may be administered or used as a necessary medical countermeasure under an EUA or IND issued by the FDA when such use is associated with a force health protection program and only if compliant with the regulatory requirements set forth below and with the approval of the Assistant Secretary of Defense for Health Affairs (ASD(HA)).

A drug or biological product may be administered for a use not described in the labeling based on standard medical practice in the United States. "Standard medical practice" refers to the authority of an individual health-care practitioner to prescribe or administer any legally marketed medical product to a patient for any condition or disease within a legitimate health care practitioner-patient relationship. These instances fall outside of a DoD force health protection program.

FDA regulatory requirements for INDs and EUAs apply to medical care provided to military and civilian DoD health-care beneficiaries located both CONUS and OCONUS.

INVESTIGATIONAL NEW DRUGS (IND)

INDs are drugs or biological products subject to FDA regulations at 21 CFR 312 and include

- A drug not approved or a biological product not licensed by the US Food and Drug Administration (FDA)
    - These products do not yet have permission from the FDA to be legally marketed and sold in the United States ("unapproved product")
    - Includes entirely new drugs, vaccines, or therapeutics which have never been licensed by the FDA for any human use
- Drug unapproved for its applied use ("off-label") These are already FDA-approved drugs or licensed biological products administered for a use not described in the FDA-approved labeling of the drug or biological product ("unapproved use of an approved product")

EMERGENCY USE AUTHORIZATION (EUA)

EUA is a special authority under US federal law. The FDA issues an EUA to allow the use of an "unapproved medical product" or an "unapproved use of an approved medical product" during a declared emergency by the Secretary of Health and Human Services (DHHS) involving a heightened risk of attack on the public or military forces.

Recent examples of using medical products under an EUA come from the medical response to the 2009 H1N1 pandemic influenza. The declaration of emergency issued by the Secretary of DHHS justified the authorization of the emergency use of certain approved neuraminidase antivirals for unapproved uses (i.e., Oseltamivir and Zanamivir) and use of an unapproved antiviral drug, peramivir.

Another example was the authorization of the emergency use of in vitro diagnostics for detection of 2009 H1N1 influenza virus . This EUA impacted DoD due to using these diagnostics on our deployed Joint Biological Agent Identification Diagnostic System (JBIADS) platforms in theater.

Refer to the FDA's online materials for further guidance on "Emergency Use Authorization of Medical Products."

REGULATORY REQUIREMENTS FOR USING INDS AND PRODUCTS UNDER AN EUA

IND medical products s are subject to FDA regulations at Part 312 of Title 21, Code of Federal Regulations, as amended, and for all military users, DoD Instruction (DODI) 6200.02 series.

Using products under an EUA for a force health protection program are subject to DODI 6200.02, section 564 of the Federal Food, Drug, and

Cosmetic Act [21 USC], sections 1107 and 1107a of title 10, USC and applicable FDA requirements.

DODI 6200.02 provides DoD policy and assigns responsibility for compliance with all federal regulations (United States Code, Executive Order, Code of Federal Regulations) for application of FDA rules to force health protection programs of the DoD involving medical products required to be used under an IND application and an EUA.

RESPONSIBILITIES FOR THE DOD FORCE HEALTH PROTECTION IND/EUA PROGRAMS

Assistant Secretary of Defense for Health Affairs (ASD(HA))

- Provides policy for the use of INDs and products under an EUA
- Reviews the rationale and justification for all DoD EUA and IND applications and provides approval prior to transmittal to the FDA
- Through the Secretary of Defense, may request that the Secretary, DHHS, declare an emergency justifying the authorization to use a medical product under an EUA as part of a force health protection program based on the determination that a military emergency, or a significant potential for a military emergency, exists involving a heightened risk to US military forces of attack with a specified biological, chemical, radiological, or nuclear agent or agents

Secretary of the Army

- Designated lead component for oversight of the use of unapproved medical products under an EUA or IND status
- The sponsor for all DoD IND protocols and use of medical products under an EUA is the US Army Surgeon General, whose representative is the US Army Medical Materiel Development Activity (USAMMDA)
- The US Army Medical Research and Materiel Command (USAMRMC) Human Subjects Research Review Board (HSRRB) reviews and approves IND protocols

Force Health Protection Division, USAMMDA (FHP/USAMMDA)

- Manages DoD's Force Health Protection (FHP) IND program
- Synchronizes, integrates, and coordinates regulatory submissions to the FDA and develops medical protocols for all the DoD Components

- Plans, implements, and sustains DoD-directed FHP IND protocols
- Provides IND medical support for military personnel exposed to CBRNE events and diseases endemic to the area of operation
- Manages the Specialized MEDCOM Response Capabilities Investigational New Drug/Emergency Use Authorizations (SMRC IND/EUA) teams who deploy to biological mass casualty incidents to facilitate the administration of IND/EUAs to military personnel
- Assists primary investigator (PI)/support staff in fulfillment of regulatory requirements
- Monitors regulatory files & provide guidance on maintenance of regulatory files
- Can send a product manager to your site to assist in protocol management; call FHP/USAMMDA at 301-619-1104 for support

CURRENT IND MEDICAL COUNTERMEASURES

Current medical countermeasures administered as INDs by FHP/USAMMDA include vaccines, drugs, and immunoglobulins to prevent and/or treat diseases caused by Category A biothreat agents, such as anthrax, botulism and smallpox. Examples of drugs or biologics that might possibly be used as INDs in the medical management of biological casualties include

- Tularemia LVS vaccine. The USAMRIID-LVS or Dynport-LVS (DVC-LVS) vaccines have not been licensed by the FDA and thus any use would be investigational
- Anthrax Vaccine Adsorbed (AVA, BioThrax). AVA is licensed for preexposure prevention of anthrax in adult. It would be considered an IND when used for postexposure prophylaxis of anthrax, or for use in children.
- Cidofovir. Cidofovir is licensed for treating cytomegalovirus retinitis in HIV patients, but not for treating generalized vaccinia. An individual physician could prescribe cidofovir "off-label" for a single case of generalized vaccinia. However, because this is not an FDA-licensed indication for the drug, it cannot legally be official policy (e.g., of the hospital, the DoD, etc) to treat all cases of generalized vaccinia with cidofovir. See below for details on how to obtain cidofovir in an emergency.

RECEIPT AND ADMINISTRATION OF INDS FOR MILITARY HEALTHCARE PROVIDERS

If an IND drug or biological product protocol exists already, call USAMRIID to discuss the case with the on-call medical officer who is familiar with the protocols for administration of IND products (1-888-USA-RIID during duty hours; DSN: 343-2257 or 301-619-2257 during non-duty hours to reach the 24-hour security desk). If the use of the IND is indicated, USAMRIID will coordinate with USAMMDA for shipping the medical product

There are several available options to determine who will administer the IND product and where

- Designate an investigator for the IND at the requesting site The proposed investigator must meet eligibility criteria (GCP training, signed FDA form 1572 and copy of protocol, etc...) and be approved by the sponsor. This can be arranged through USAMMDA
- DoD has pre-trained, designated investigators who are already established at several of the major MEDCENs who could potentially travel to the patient to administer the IND product Alternatively, the patient could be evacuated to the nearest medical center with a pre-trained, designated investigator who will administer the product
- USAMMDA has previously designated certain qualified individuals to serve on a specialized MEDCOM Response Capabilities IND/EUA (SMRC IND/EUA) teams to administer IND products For large numbers of casualties, or the need for a time-critical IND administration, USAMMDA might consider sending a SMRC IND/EUA team to run the protocol and administer the IND product

If no satisfactory FDA-approved medical product is available for a medical countermeasure against a particular threat at the time of need under a force health protection program, request approval by the ASD(HA) to use an unapproved product under an EUA or, if an EUA is not feasible, under an IND application (DODI 6200.02 series applies)

PROCESS FOR OBTAINING CIDOFOVIR AND VIG-IV

VIG-IV is a FDA-licensed medical product and is no longer administered under an IND protocol for treatment of specific smallpox vaccine adverse reactions

Cidofovir (Vistide®) is licensed to treat cytomegalvirus (CMV) retinitis (a serious eye infection) in HIV-infected people. It is not licensed to treat adverse reactions caused by smallpox vaccine (e.g., generalized vaccinia, eczema vaccinatum, progressive vaccinia) so it can only be used "off-label" (prescribed by a physician to treat a condition for which it has not been specifically approved) or through an IND protocol.

Cidofovir is available through the CDC under IND protocol for treatment of specific smallpox vaccine adverse reactions. VIG-IV is recommended as the first line of therapy. Under the IND, cidofovir may be considered as a secondary treatment only in consultation with HHS/CDC and when VIG-IV is not efficacious.

Cidofovir is released from the CDC and will be shipped by the CDC Strategic National Stockpile (SNS). The cost of cidofovir and the cost of shipping will be covered by the US Government. Arrival of shipments should be expected within 12 hours of the approval for release.

The cidofovir IND protocol mandates that the treating physician must become a co-investigator primarily responsible for completing follow-up forms describing the clinical status of the patient being treated with cidofovir, including the prompt report of any significant adverse reaction in the recipient. Detailed information on the requirements of the IND will be shipped with the products.

Military Health Care Providers: VIG-IV stocks have been prepositioned for DOD in CONUS and OCONUS Contact your DoD Regional Vaccine Healthcare Centers (VHC) office during normal business hours or the DoD VHC Network's Vaccine Clinical Call Center 24/7 at 1-866-210-6469 for the most current process for obtaining VIG-IV.

Military clinicians requesting use of cidofovir must consult with an infectious disease or allergy-immunology specialist. Consultations will be arranged via the DoD Vaccine Healthcare Centers (VHC) Network's Vaccine Clinical Call Center (866-210-6469) who will notify the Military Vaccine Agency (MILVAX) of case specifics.

The infectious disease or allergy-immunology specialist physician, in consultation with the VHC, will contact the CDC Director's Emergency Operations Center (DEOC) at 770-488-7100 and consult with on-call staff in the Division of Bioterrorism and Response (BDPR). The CDC is the release authority for cidofovir under an IND protocol and will coordinate release of this medical product from the CDC's Strategic National Stockpile (SNS).

Civilian Health Care Providers: Civilian health-care providers should first contact their state health department when seeking consultation for civilian patients experiencing a severe or unexpected adverse event after smallpox vaccination or when requesting cidofovir. If further consultation is required, or cidofovir is recommended, the physician and state health department can request consultation through the CDC Director's Emergency Operations Center as above.

PROCESS FOR OBTAINING BOTULINUM ANTITOXIN UNDER IND

In 2010, CDC announced the availability of a new heptavalent botulinum antitoxin (HBAT, Cangene Corporation) through a CDC-sponsored FDA IND protocol. HBAT replaced a licensed bivalent botulinum antitoxin AB and an investigational monovalent botulinum antitoxin E (BAT-AB and BAT-E, Sanofi Pasteur) with expiration of these products in March 2010. HBAT is the only botulinum antitoxin currently available in the US for naturally occurring noninfant botulism and is available only from the CDC.

All medical-care providers who suspect a diagnosis of botulism in a patient should immediately call their state health department's emergency 24-hour telephone number The state health department will contact the CDC DEOC (770-488-7100) to report suspected botulism cases, arrange for a clinical consultation by telephone and, if indicated, request release of HBAT. The CDC DEOC will then contact the on-call Foodborne and Diarrheal Diseases Branch medical officer.

BabyBIG® (botulism immune globulin) remains available for infant botulism through the California Infant Botulism Treatment and Prevention Program. BabyBIG® is an orphan drug that consists of human-derived botulism antitoxin antibodies and is approved by FDA for the treatment of infant botulism types A and B. To obtain BabyBIG® for suspected infant botulism, the patient's physician must contact the Infant Botulism Treatment and Prevention Program (IBTPP) on-call physician at (510) 231-7600 to review the indications for such treatment.

APPENDIX M: USE OF DRUGS/VACCINES IN SPECIAL OR VULNERABLE POPULATIONS IN THE CONTEXT OF BIOTERRORISM

(The pediatric patient, nursing mothers, pregnant patient, and the immunocompromised)

PEDIATRIC PATIENTS

Management of pediatric patients exposed to biowarfare agents may be problematic for several reasons. Some antimicrobials and vaccines are not licensed for use in children. Additionally, most investigational new drug (IND) applications do not include children in their subject groups. For example, the Anthrax Vaccine (AVA) is licensed only for preexposure use in people aged 18-65. While AVA may be effective in preventing anthrax in children as well, it has not been studied in pediatric populations. Smallpox vaccine can be used only in patients 6 months of age or older.

Some vaccines, even though licensed for use in children, are more problematic in children than in adults. Smallpox vaccine is much more likely to lead to postvaccinial encephalitis, an often-fatal condition, when given to young children. Yellow fever vaccine is more likely to cause severe encephalitis in young infants than it is in adults.

Some antimicrobials are relatively contraindicated in children due to real or perceived risks which do not appear to be present in adult populations. Tetracyclines and fluoroquinolones are the two classes of antibiotics that generate the most concern as they are the drugs of choice for treating or preventing many biowarfare diseases.

Tetracyclines This class of antibiotics is generally contraindicated in children less than 8 years old because the antibiotic and its pigmented breakdown products can cause permanent dental staining and, more rarely, enamel hypoplasia during odontogenesis. The degree of staining is proportional to the total dose received and is thus dependent upon both dose and duration of therapy. Thus, doxycycline, which is given only twice per day, represents a lower risk than other tetracyclines. Tetracyclines may also cause reversible delay in bone growth rate during the course of therapy. Despite these relative contraindications, the American Academy of

Pediatrics (AAP) recommends tetracyclines for treating certain severe illnesses that respond poorly to other antibiotics (e.g., Rocky Mountain spotted fever and other rickettsial diseases), specifically including treatment or prevention of anthrax disease.

Fluoroquinolones This class of antibiotics is generally contraindicated in patients less than 18-years old because it is associated with cartilage damage in juvenile animal models. While sporadic cases of arthropathy in humans have been reported, they have primarily been associated with adults and children receiving perfloxacin, a fluoroquinolone commonly used in France. Ciprofloxacin, which has been used extensively in children, has not thus far been associated with arthropathy and seems to be well tolerated. For this reason, the AAP recognizes that fluoroquinolones may be used in children in special circumstances, specifically including treating or preventing anthrax. In fact, ciprofloxacin is specifically licensed by the FDA for postexposure prophylaxis against anthrax IN CHILDREN.

General guidance In pediatric cases of suspected biowarfare exposure or disease in which the empiric treatment of choice is a drug with limited pediatric experience, one may be left with few viable alternatives than to treat with such a drug. For example, if a 5-year-old child is suspected to have been exposed to an aerosol of *Bacillus anthracis* of unknown antibiotic susceptibility, the best initial choice of antibiotic may be ciprofloxacin or doxycycline (In fact, for this reason, the FDA and AAP recommend either of these drugs for empiric postexposure prophylaxis of inhalational anthrax). If the organism is later determined to be susceptible to penicillins, then one could switch to amoxicillin to complete the course of antibiotics. If the organism is not susceptible to penicillin but is susceptible to doxycycline and ciprofloxacin, then ciprofloxacin may represent a better choice for continued prophylaxis, as arthropathy from fluoroquinolones thus far has proved rare in children, whereas the necessarily prolonged course of doxycycline (perhaps 60 days) could lead to significant dental staining. If the same child was exposed to *Yersinia pestis* susceptible to both ciprofloxacin and doxycycline, doxycycline might be an equally good choice as ciprofloxacin, as the short (7 day) course of postexposure prophylaxis is unlikely to result in dental staining. Clinicians must use judgment in these cases, taking into account the organism's antibiotic susceptibilities, the available prophylaxis or treatment options, and the risk versus benefit to the individual patient. Antimicrobial doses are often different in children, and prescribed according to patient weight. Some representative antibiotics and their pediatric doses are included in Table 1.

NURSING MOTHERS

Some medications are excreted in breast milk (see Table 1), and thus may be ingested by nursing infants. Such medications, if contraindicated in infants and orally absorbed, should also be avoided by breast-feeding mothers if possible. It is generally recommended that fluoroquinolones, tetracyclines, and chloramphenicol be avoided in nursing mothers. Obviously, these drugs may represent the treatment of choice for many biowarfare agents; thus, practitioners must again weigh the risks of administering these drugs with the potential adverse consequences of using a less effective medication. In some cases, temporary cessation of nursing while on the offending drug may be necessary. Antibiotics generally considered safe during nursing are aminoglycosides, penicillins, cephalosporins, and macrolides.

PREGNANT PATIENTS

Some medications that are useful and safe for treating diseases in women may nonetheless pose specific risks during pregnancy. FDA has developed the following pregnancy risk categories. **A**: studies in pregnant women show no risk; **B**: animal studies show no risk but human studies are not adequate or animal toxicity has been shown but human studies show no risk; **C**: animal studies show toxicity, human studies are inadequate but benefit of use may exceed risk; **D**: evidence of human risk but benefits may outweigh risks; **X**: fetal abnormalities in humans, risk outweighs benefit. Pregnancy risk categories for representative therapeutics are included in Table 1.

Again, tetracyclines and fluoroquinolones must be addressed, as they are empiric treatments of choice for many biowarfare diseases yet relatively contraindicated in pregnancy. Animal studies indicate that tetracyclines can retard skeletal development in the fetus; embryotoxicity has also been described in animals treated early in pregnancy. There are few adequate studies of fluoroquinolones in pregnant women; existing published data, albeit sparse, do not demonstrate a substantial teratogenic risk associated with ciprofloxacin use during pregnancy. In cases for which either ciprofloxacin or doxycycline are recommended for initial empiric prophylaxis (e.g., inhalational anthrax, plague, or tularemia), ciprofloxacin, if tolerated, may represent the lower risk option; then, after antibiotic susceptibility data are gained, antibiotics should be switched to lower risk alternatives if possible.

While most vaccinations are to be avoided during pregnancy, killed vaccines are generally considered to be of low risk. While live vaccines (e.g., measles-mumps-rubella) are contraindicated during pregnancy, a notable exception is the administration of the smallpox vaccine (vaccinia) to pregnant women after a known or highly suspected exposure to the smallpox virus during an outbreak.

THE IMMUNOCOMPROMISED PATIENT

While immunocompromised individuals may be more susceptible to biowarfare disease or may develop more severe disease than immunocompetent patients, consensus groups generally recommend using the same antimicrobial regimens recommended for their immunocompetent counterparts. The most obvious difference in management of these patients concerns receipt of live vaccines, such as the currently licensed smallpox vaccine, or the LVS tularemia vaccine. Generally, it is best to manage these individuals on a case-by-case basis and in concert with immunologists and/or infectious disease specialists.

TABLE 1. Antimicrobials in Special Populations

Class of Drug	Pregnancy category	Drug name	breast milk	Pediatric Oral Dose	Pediatric parenteral dose
Aminoglycosides	C	Gentamicin	(+) small		3-7.5 mg/kg/day in 3 doses (IV or IM)
	D	Amikacin	(+) small		15-22.5 mg/kg/day in 3 doses (max 1.5g/day) (IV or IM)
	D	Streptomycin	(+) small		30 mg/kg/day in 2 doses (max 2g/day) (IM only)
	D	Tobramycin	(+) small		3-7.5 mg/kg/day in 3 doses (IV or IM)
Carbapenems	C	Imipenem	(?)		60 mg/kg/day in 4 doses (max 4g/day) (IV or IM)
	B	Meropenem	(?)		60-120 mg/kg/day in 3 doses (max 6g/day) (IV)
Cephalosporins	B	Cefriaxone	(+) trace		80 - 100 mg/kg in 1 or 2 doses (max 4g/day) (IV or IM)
	B	Ceftazidime	(+) trace		125-150 mg/kg/day in 3 doses (max 6g/day) (IV or IM)
	B	Cephalexin	(+) trace	25-50 mg/kg/day in 3-4 doses	
	B	Cefuroxime	(+) trace	20-30 mg/kg/day in 2 doses (max 2g/day)	100-150 mg/kg/day in 3 doses (max 6g/day) (IV or IM)
	B	Cefepime	(+) trace		150mg in 3 doses (max 4g/day) (IV or IM)
Chloramphenicol	C		(+)	50-100 mg/kg/day in 4 doses (formulation not avail in US)	50-100 mg/kg/day in 4 doses (max 4g/day) (IV)
Fluoroquinolones	C	Ciprofloxacin	(+)	30 mg/kg/day in 2 doses (max 1.5g)	20-30 mg/kg/day in 2 doses (max 800mg/day) (IV)

Class of Drug	Pregnancy category	Drug name	breast milk	Pediatric Oral Dose	Pediatric parenteral dose
Glycopeptides	C	Vancomycin	(+)		40-60 mg/kg/day in 4 doses (max 4g/day) (IV)
Lincos-amides	B	Clindamycin	(+)	10-20 mg/kg/day in 3-4 doses (max 1.8g/day)	25-40 mg/kg/day in 3-4 doses (max 2.7g/day) (IV or IM)
Lipopeptides	B	Daptomycin	(?)		4 mg/kg once daily (IV)
Macrolides	B	Azithrothromycin	(+)	5-12 mg/kg/day once daily (max 600mg/day)	
	C	Clarithromycin	(?)	15 mg/kg/day in 2 doses (max 1g/day)	
	B	Erythromycin	(+)	30-50 mg/kg/day in 2-4 doses (max 2g/day)	15-50 mg/kg/day in 4 doses (max 4g/day) (IV)
Mono-bactams	B	Aztreonam	(+)trace		90-120 mg/kg/day in 3-4 doses (max 8g) (IV or IM)
Oxalodi-nones	C	Linezolid	(+)	20-30 mg/kg/day in 3 doses (max 800/mg/day)	20-30 mg/kg/day in 3 doses (max 1200/mg/day) (IV)
Penicillins	B	Amoxicillin	(+) trace	25-9 0mg/kg/day in 3 doses (max 1.5g/day)	
	B	Ampicillin	(+) trace	50-100 mg/kg/day in 4 doses (max 4g/day)	200-400 mg/kg/day in 4 doses (max 12g/day) (IV or IM)
	B	Penicillin G	(+) trace		25000-400000U/kg/day in 4-6 doses (max 24milU/day) (IV or IM)
	B	Nafcillin	(+) trace		100-150 mg/kg/day in 4 doses (max12g) (IV or IM)

Class of Drug	Pregnancy category	Drug name	breast milk	Pediatric Oral Dose	Pediatric parenteral dose
Rifampin	C		(+)	10-20 mg/kg/day in 1-2 doses (max 600mg/day)	10-20 mg/kg/day in 1-2 doses (max 600mg/day)
Strepto-gramins	B	Dalfopristin-Quinupristin	(+)		22.5 mg/kg/day in 3 doses (IV)
Sulfon-amides	C	Trimethoprim/ Sulfamethoxa-zole	(+) trace	8-12 mg/kg/day TMP in 4 doses (max 320 mg/day TMP)	8-12 mg/kg/day TMP in 4 doses (IV)
Tetracyclines	D	Doxycycline	(+)	2-4 mg/kg/day in 1-2 doses (max 200mg/day)	2-4 mg/kg/day in 1-2 doses (max 200mg/day)(IV)
	D	Tetracycline	(+)	20-50 mg/kg/day in 4 doses (max 2g)	10-25 mg/kg/day in 2-4 doses (max 2g) (IV)
Cidofovir	C		(?)		5mg/kg once with probenecid and hydration
Oseltamivir	C		(+)	1-12 years old: $\leq$15 kg: 30 mg twice daily; 15-23 kg: 45 mg 2X/day; 23-40kg: 60mg 2X/day; >40kg: adult dose	
Ribavirin	X		(?)	30 mg/kg once, then 15 mg/kg/day in 2 doses (VHFs)	Same as for adults, dosed by weight (IV)

Note: (1) The above dose are for children outside of the neonatal period Neonatal doses may be different

Note: (2) Pediatric antibiotic doses included in this table represent generic doses for severe disease. They may not accurately reflect expert consensus for treatment of some specific BW diseases (anthrax, plague, tularemia). For those diseases, refer to the specific chapter for recommendations.

APPENDIX N: EMERGENCY RESPONSE CONTACTS FBI & PUBLIC HEALTH

Federal Bureau of Investigation (FBI) Field Offices (by state)

Alabama

FBI Birmingham
1000 18th Street North
Birmingham, AL 35203
birmingham.fbi.gov
(205) 326-6166

FBI Mobile
200 N. Royal Street
Mobile, AL 36602
mobile.fbi.gov
(251) 438-3674

Alaska

FBI Anchorage
101 East Sixth Avenue
Anchorage, AK 99501-2524
anchorage.fbi.gov
907-276-4441

Arizona

FBI Phoenix
Suite 400
201 East Indianola Avenue
Phoenix, AZ 85012-2080
phoenix.fbi.gov
(602) 279-5511

Arkansas

FBI Little Rock
#24 Shackleford West Boulevard
Little Rock, AR 72211-3755
littlerock.fbi.gov
(501) 221-9100

California

FBI Los Angeles
Suite 1700, FOB
11000 Wilshire Boulevard
Los Angeles, CA 90024-3672
losangeles.fbi.gov
(310) 477-6565

FBI Sacramento
4500 Orange Grove Avenue
Sacramento, CA 95841-4205
sacramento.fbi.gov
(916) 481-9110

FBI San Diego
Federal Office Building
9797 Aero Drive
San Diego, CA 92123-1800
sandiego.fbi.gov
(858) 565-1255

FBI San Francisco
450 Golden Gate Avenue, 13th. Floor
San Francisco, CA 94102-9523
sanfrancisco.fbi.gov
(415) 553-7400

Colorado

FBI Denver
8000 East 36th Avenue
Denver, CO 80238
denver.fbi.gov
(303) 629-7171

Connecticut

FBI New Haven
600 State Street
New Haven, CT 06511-6505
newhaven.fbi.gov
(203) 777-6311

District of Columbia

FBI Washington
Washington Metropolitan Field Office
601 4th Street, N.W.
Washington, D.C. 20535-0002
washingtondc.fbi.gov
(202) 278-2000

Florida

FBI Jacksonville
6061 Gate Parkway
Jacksonville, FL 32256
jacksonville.fbi.gov
(904) 248-7000

FBI North Miami Beach
16320 Northwest Second Avenue
North Miami Beach, FL 33169-6508
miami.fbi.gov
(305) 944-9101

FBI Tampa
5525 West Gray Street
Tampa, FL 33609
tampa.fbi.gov
(813) 253-1000

Georgia

FBI Atlanta
Suite 400
2635 Century Parkway, Northeast
Atlanta, GA 30345-3112
atlanta.fbi.gov
(404) 679-9000

Hawaii

FBI Honolulu
Room 4-230,
Prince Kuhio FOB
300 Ala Moana Boulevard
Honolulu, HI 96813
honolulu.fbi.gov
(808) 566-4300

Illinois

FBI Chicago
2111 West Roosevelt Road Chicago, IL
60608-1128
chicago.fbi.gov
(312) 421-6700

FBI Springfield
900 East Linton Avenue
Springfield, IL 62703
springfield.fbi.gov
(217) 522-9675

Indiana

FBI Indianapolis
Room 679, FOB
575 North Pennsylvania Street
Indianapolis, IN 46204-1585
indianapolis.fbi.gov
(317) 639-3301

Kentucky

FBI Louisville
12401 Sycamore Station Place
Louisville , KY
40299-6198
louisville.fbi.gov
(502) 263-6000

Louisiana

FBI New Orleans
2901 Leon C. Simon Dr.
New Orleans, LA 70126
neworleans.fbi.gov
(504) 816-3000

Maryland

FBI Baltimore
2600 Lord Baltimore Drive
Baltimore, MD 21244
baltimore.fbi.gov
(410) 265-8080

Massachusetts

FBI Boston
Suite 600
One Center Plaza
Boston, MA 02108
boston.fbi.gov
(617) 742-5533

Michigan

FBI Detroit
26th. Floor, P. V. McNamara FOB
477 Michigan Avenue
Detroit, MI 48226
detroit.fbi.gov
(313) 965-2323

Minnesota

FBI Minneapolis
Suite 1100
111 Washington Avenue, South
Minneapolis, MN 55401-2176
minneapolis.fbi.gov
(612) 376-3200

Mississippi

FBI Jackson
1220 Echelon Parkway
Jackson, MS 39213
jackson.fbi.gov
(601) 948-5000

Missouri

FBI Kansas City
1300 Summit
Kansas City, MO 64105-1362
kansascity.fbi.gov
(816) 512-8200

FBI St. Louis
2222 Market Street
St. Louis, MO 63103-2516
stlouis.fbi.gov
(314) 231-4324

Nebraska

FBI Omaha
4411 South 121st Court
Omaha, NE 68137-2112
omaha.fbi.gov
(402) 493-8688

Nevada

FBI Las Vegas
John Lawrence Bailey Building
1787 West Lake Mead Boulevard
Las Vegas, NV 89106-2135
lasvegas.fbi.gov
(702) 385-1281

New Jersey

FBI Newark
11 Centre Place
Newark, NJ 07102-9889
newark.fbi.gov
(973) 792-3000

New Mexico

FBI Albuquerque
4200 Luecking Park Ave. NE
Albuquerque, NM 87107
albuquerque.fbi.gov
(505) 889-1300

New York

FBI Albany
200 McCarty Avenue
Albany, NY 12209
albany.fbi.gov
(518) 465-7551

FBI Buffalo
One FBI Plaza
Buffalo, NY 14202-2698
buffalo.fbi.gov
(716) 856-7800

FBI New York
26 Federal Plaza, 23rd. Floor
New York, NY 10278-0004
newyork.fbi.gov
(212) 384-1000

North Carolina

FBI Charlotte
7915 Microsoft Way
Charlotte, NC 28273
charlotte.fbi.gov
(704) 672-6100

Ohio

FBI Cincinnati
Room 9000
550 Main Street
Cincinnati, OH 45202-8501
cincinnati.fbi.gov
(513) 421-4310

FBI Cleveland
Federal Office Building
1501 Lakeside Avenue
Cleveland, OH 44114
cleveland.fbi.gov
(216) 522-1400

Oklahoma

FBI Oklahoma City
3301 West Memorial Drive
Oklahoma City, OK 73134
oklahomacity.fbi.gov
(405) 290-7770

Oregon

FBI Portland
Suite 400, Crown Plaza Building
1500 Southwest 1st Avenue
Portland, OR 97201-5828
portland.fbi.gov
(503) 224-4181

Pennsylvania

FBI Philadelphia
8th. Floor
William J. Green Jr. FOB
600 Arch Street
Philadelphia, PA 19106
philadelphia.fbi.gov
(215) 418-4000

FBI Pittsburgh
3311 East Carson St.
Pittsburgh, PA 15203
pittsburgh.fbi.gov
(412) 432-4000

Puerto Rico

FBI San Juan
Room 526, U.S. Federal Bldg.
150 Carlos Chardon Avenue
Hato Rey
San Juan, PR 00918-1716
sanjuan.fbi.gov
(787) 754-6000

South Carolina

FBI Columbia
151 Westpark Blvd
Columbia, SC 29210-3857
columbia.fbi.gov
(803) 551-4200

Tennessee

FBI Knoxville
1501 Dowell Springs Boulevard
Knoxville, TN 37909
knoxville.fbi.gov
(865) 544-0751

FBI Memphis
Suite 3000, Eagle Crest Bldg.
225 North Humphreys Blvd.
Memphis, TN 38120-2107
memphis.fbi.gov
(901) 747-4300

Texas

FBI Dallas
One Justice Way
Dallas, Texas 75220
dallas.fbi.gov
(972) 559-5000

FBI El Paso
660 S. Mesa Hills Drive
El Paso, Texas 79912-5533
elpaso.fbi.gov
(915) 832-5000

FBI Houston
1 Justice Park Drive
Houston, TX 77092
houston.fbi.gov
(713) 693-5000

FBI San Antonio
5740 University Heights Boulevard
San Antonio, TX 78249
sanantonio.fbi.gov
(210) 225-6741

Utah

FBI Salt Lake City
Suite 1200, 257 Towers Bldg.
257 East, 200 South
Salt Lake City, UT 84111-2048
saltlakecity.fbi.gov
(801) 579-1400

Virginia

FBI Norfolk
150 Corporate Boulevard
Norfolk, VA 23502-4999
norfolk.fbi.gov
(757) 455-0100

FBI Richmond
1970 E. Parham Road
Richmond, VA 23228
richmond.fbi.gov
(804) 261-1044
For Northern Virginia, contact the Washington Field Office.

Washington

FBI Seattle
1110 Third Avenue
Seattle, WA 98101-2904
seattle.fbi.gov
(206) 622-0460

Wisconsin

FBI Milwaukee
Suite 600
330 East Kilbourn Avenue
Milwaukee, WI 53202-6627
milwaukee.fbi.gov
(414) 276-4684

State Health Departments (by state)

Alabama

Department of Public Health
The RSA Tower
201 Monroe Street
Montgomery, Alabama 36104
334-206-5300
1-800-ALA-1818
www.adph.org

Alaska

Division of Public Health
350 Main Street, Room 508
Juneau, Alaska 99801
(907) 465-3090
Fax: (907) 465-4632
http://health.hss.state.ak.us

Arizona

Department of Health Services
150 North 18th Avenue
Phoenix, Arizona 85007
(602) 542-1025
Fax: (602) 542-0883
http://www.azdhs.gov

Arkansas

Department of Health
4815 West Markham Street
Little Rock, Arkansas 72205
1-501-661-2000 or 1-800-462-0599
www.healthy.arkansas.gov

California

Department of Public Health
(916) 558-1784
http://www.cdph.ca.gov

Colorado

Department of Public Health and Environment

4300 Cherry Creek Drive South
Denver, Colorado 80246-1530
303- 692-2000
1-800-886-7689 (In-state)
http://www.cdphe.state.co.us/

Connecticut

Department of Public Health

410 Capitol Avenue Hartford, CT 06134
Phone: 860-509-8000
http://www.ct.gov/dph/

Delaware

Division of Public Health

417 Federal Street
Jesse Cooper Building
Dover, DE 19901
(302) 744-4700
FAX: (302) 739-6659
http://www.dhss.delaware.gov/dhss/dph/

District of Columbia

Department of Health

899 North Capitol Street, NE
Washington, DC 20002
(202) 442-5955
http://dchealth.dc.gov/doh/

Florida

Department of Health

2585 Merchants Row Boulevard Tallahassee, Florida 32399
(850) 245-4444
http://www.doh.state.fl.us/

Georgia

Department of Public Health

Two Peachtree Street, NW
Atlanta, Georgia 30303-3186
Phone: (404) 657-2700
http://health.state.ga.us/

Hawaii

Department of Public Health

Kinau Hale
1250 Punchbowl Street
Honolulu, HI 96813
(808) 586-4400
http://hawaii.gov/health

Idaho

Department of Health and Welfare

P.O. Box 83720
Boise, ID 83720-0036
(208) 334-5500
http://www.healthandwelfare.idaho.gov/

Illinois

Department of Public Health

535 West Jefferson Street
Springfield, Illinois 62761
217-782-4977
Fax 217-782-3987
http://www.idph.state.il.us/

Indiana

State Department of Health

2 North Meridian Street
Indianapolis, IN 46204
(317) 233-1325
http://www.state.in.us/isdh/

Iowa

Department of Public Health

321 E. 12th Street
Des Moines, Iowa, 50319-0075
(515) 281-7689
toll-free at 1-866-227-9878
http://www.idph.state.ia.us/

Kansas

Department of Health and Environment

Curtis State Office Building
1000 SW Jackson
Topeka, Kansas 66612
785-296-1500
http://www.kdheks.gov/

Kentucky

Department for Public Health

275 East Main Street
Frankfort, KY 40621
(502) 564-3970
http://chfs.ky.gov/dph/

Louisiana

Department of Health and Hospitals

P.O. Box 629
Baton Rouge, LA 70821-0629
(225) 342-9500

Maine

Department of Health and Human Services

221 State Street
Augusta, ME 04333
207-287-3707
Fax 207-287-3005
http://www.maine.gov/dhhs/

Maryland

201 West Preston Street
Baltimore, MD 21201
(410) 767-6500 or 1-877-463-3464
http://www.dhmh.state.md.us/

Maryland

Department of Health and Mental Hygene

201 West Preston Street
Baltimore, MD 21201
(401) 767-6500 or 1-877-463-3463
http://www.dhmh.state.md.us/

Massachusetts

Department of Public Health

250 Washington Street
Boston, Massachusetts 02108
http://www.mass.gov/

Michigan

Department of Community Health

Capitol View Building
201 Townsend Street
Lansing, Michigan 48913
517-373-3740
http://www.michigan.gov/mdch/

Minnesota

Department of Health

P.O. Box 64975
St. Paul, MN 55164-0975
651-201-5000
888-345-0823
http://www.health.state.mn.us/

Mississippi

State Department of Health

570 East Woodrow Wilson Drive
Jackson, MS 39216
601-576-7400
1-866-458-4948
http://msdh.ms.gov/index.htm

Missouri

Department of Health and Senior Services

912 Wildwood
P.O. Box 570
Jefferson City, Missouri 65102
Phone: 573-751-6400
Fax: 573-751-6010
Email: info@health.mo.gov
http://health.mo.gov/

Montana

Department of Public Health and Human Services

111 North Sanders, Room 301
Helena, MT 59620
(406) 444-5622
Fax: (406) 444-1970
http://www.dphhs.mt.gov/

Nebraska

Department of Health & Human Services

301 Centennial Mall South
Lincoln, Nebraska 68509
(402) 471-3121
http://www.hhs.state.ne.us/

Nevada

Department of Health & Human Services

4126 Technology Way, Suite 100
Carson City, Nevada 89706-2009
(775) 684-4000
(775) 684-4010 Fax
http://dhhs.nv.gov/

New Hampshire

Division of Public Health Services

NH Department of Health & Human Services
29 Hazen Drive
Concord, NH 03301
(603) 271-4501
(800) 852-3345 Ext. 4501
http://www.dhhs.nh.gov/dphs/

New Jersey

Department of Health and Senior Services

P. O. Box 360, Trenton, NJ 08625-0360
Phone: (609) 292-7837
Toll-free in NJ: 1-800-367-6543
http://www.state.nj.us/health/

New Mexico

Department of Health

1190 South St. Francis Drive
Santa Fe, NM 87502
Phone: (505) 827-2613
FAX: (505) 827-2530
http://nmhealth.org/

New York State

Department of Health

Corning Tower
Empire State Plaza,
Albany, NY 12237
Public Health Duty Officer Helpline
1-866-881-2809
http://www.health.state.ny.us/

North Carolina

Division of Public Health

1931 Mail Service Center
Raleigh, NC 27699-1931
919-707-5000
Fax: 919-870-4829
http://publichealth.nc.gov/

North Dakota

Department of Health

600 East Boulevard Avenue
Bismarck, N.D. 58505-0200
701.328.2372
Fax: 701.328.4727
http://www.ndhealth.gov/

Ohio

Department of Health

246 N. High St.
Columbus, Ohio 43215
(614) 466-3543
mailto:Director@odh.ohio.gov
http://www.odh.ohio.gov/

Oklahoma

State Department of Health

1000 NE 10th
Oklahoma City, OK 73117
(405)271-5600
1-800-522-0203
http://www.ok.gov/health/

Oregon

Public Health Division

800 NE Oregon Street
Portland, OR 97232
971-673-1222
Fax: 971-673-1299
http://public.health.oregon.gov/

Pennsylvania

Department of Health

Health and Welfare Building
8th Floor West
625 Forster Street
Harrisburg, PA 17120
1-877-724-3258
http://www.portal.state.pa.us/portal/server.pt/community/department_of_health_home/

Rhode Island

Department of Health

3 Capitol Hill
Providence, RI 02908
(401) 222-5960
http://www.health.ri.gov/

South Carolina

Department of Health and Environmental Control

2600 Bull Street
Columbia, SC 29201
(803) 898-DHEC (3432)
http://www.scdhec.gov/

South Dakota

Department of Health

600 East Capitol Ave.
Pierre, SD 57501-2536
(605) 773-3361
1-800-738-2301 (in state)
http://doh.sd.gov/

Tennessee

Department of Health

425 5th Avenue North
Cordell Hull Building, 3rd Floor
Nashville, TN 37243
(615) 741-3111
http://health.state.tn.us/

Texas

Department of State Health Services

1100 West 49th Street
Austin, Texas 78756-3199
(512) 458-7111
1-888-963-7111
http://www.dshs.state.tx.us/

Utah

Department of Health

P.O. Box 141010
Salt Lake City, UT 84114-1010
801-538-6003
http://health.utah.gov/

Vermont

Department of Health

108 Cherry Street
Burlington, VT 05402
Voice: 802-863-7200
In Vermont 800-464-4343
Fax: 802-865-7754
http://healthvermont.gov/

Virginia

Department of Health

P.O. Box 2448
Richmond, Virginia 23218-2448
109 Governor Street
Richmond, Virginia 23219
(804) 864-7002
http://www.vdh.state.va.us/

Washington State

Department of Health

101 Israel Road SE
Tumwater, Washington 98501
PO BOX 47890
Olympia, Washington 98504-7890
(360) 236-4030
http://www.doh.wa.gov/

West Virginia

Department of Health and Human Resources
Bureau for Public Health

Room 702
350 Capitol Street
Charleston, WV 25301-3712
Telephone: (304) 558-2971
Fax: (304) 558-1035
http://www.wvdhhr.org/bph/

Wisconsin

Department of Health Services

1 West Wilson Street
Madison, WI 53703
608-266-1865
http://www.dhs.wisconsin.gov/

Wyoming

Department of Health

401 Hathaway Building
Cheyenne, WY 82002
(307) 777-7656
(866) 571-0944
Fax: (307) 777-7439
http://www.health.wyo.gov/

Made in the USA
Monee, IL
30 June 2022

98879648R10154